MEDICAL QUACKERY
Contraptions, Contrivances, and Gadgets

In 1796, the first U.S. patent for a medical device of dubious distinction was issued to Dr. Elisha Perkins for his Metallic Tractors, a set of dissimilar metal prods. It was (and in some circles still is) commonly believed that good health is an equilibrium of magnetic and electrical charges. Magnets and electrical devices have been applied to ailing bodies in an effort to "restore" this balance.

During the unprincipled years of the late 19th and early 20th centuries, useless pills, salves and liquid nostrums were widely hawked by pitchmen who extolled their mythical virtues. Colorful compounds--bitters, elixirs, vermifuges, pectorals, alteratives, balms, ambrocations and imaginative mechanical and electrical devices were advertised everywhere--magazines, newspapers, mail order catalogs, store fronts, fence posts and barn roofs. The Sears Roebuck catalog was a cornucopia of concoctions and contraptions. Hundreds of traveling medicine shows extolled the virtues of worthless preparations and products:

Dr. Kilmer's Swamp Root
Dr. Pierce's Golden Medical Discovery
Dr. Pierce's Nasal Douche
Kickapoo Indian Sagwa
Sarsaparilla (sasparilla)
Dr. Hercules Sanche's Oxydonor
Balm of Gilead
Rattlesnake Oil
Pulvermacher's Electro-Galvanic Chain Kidney Pads
Anodyne Cordials
Magnetic Plasters
Pink Pills for Pale People
Thayer's Slippery Elm Lozenges
Men's Secret
Swamp Oil

Galvanic Love Powder
The Invalid's Friend and Hope
Princess Lotus Blossom's Vital Sparks
Kurakoff
Wilsonia Magnetic Garments
Dr. Fahnstock's Celebrated Vermifuge
…and countless more.

The golden age of quackery took advantage of a receptive, unsophisticated public, awed by a barrage of legitimate discoveries from scientific luminaries like Edison, Bell, Marconi, Curie, Becquerel and Tesla.

During the first two decades of the 20th century, a number of radium cures were unleashed on a credulous public, unaware that Madame Curie's fingers had fallen off from radioactive exposure before her death. That particularly-potent patent medicine period ended in about 1930 when steel magnate Eben MacBurney Byers, who boasted he had drunk 1400 bottles of radium water in two years, died after his jaw fell off.

The vast majority of patent medicines were alcohol-based, many containing opium or morphine as well. Virtually none contained the ingredients they claimed to have, and none could heal. Princess Lotus Blossom's Vital Sparks, promising to revitalize masculine virility, and claimed to be "from the Quali Quah pouch of the Kup Ki See Chinese Turtle," was actually made by rolling rock candy in powdered aloe.

Tiger Fat, a cure-all balm touted to be rendered from Royal Bengal tigers' backbones, was concocted of Vaseline, camphor, menthol, eucalyptus oil, turpentine, wintergreen oil, and paraffin. Liver Pads, promoted as a cure for liver diseases, were nothing more than small fabric swatches with a spot of red pepper and glue; when the body heat melted the glue, the sting of the red pepper was perceived as a healing sensation.

During this period of medical chicanery, anyone with charisma and a horse could travel from town to town hawking their nostrums. The pitchmen had a caste system: When the "high pitch" salesmen -- elevated on a stage or wagon -- were in town , the "low pitch" salesmen who worked the streets from a "med case" or "keister" set on a portable tripod or table, were expected to fold up their wares until their superiors left town.

The nostrum peddlers commonly represented themselves as Quakers, Orientals or Indians, appearing in hundreds of traveling pageants which assembled after the Civil War. The largest medicine shows were assembled by John E. "Doc" Healy and Charles H. "Texas Charlie" Bigelow in 1881. Their 20 road shows stopped at towns across rural America to offer hours of entertainment-- singing, dancing, trained animals, minstrel shows, movies, chalk talks and skits ("afterpieces"), all for a dime. Smaller road shows were free, supported by working the crowds with medications.

A typical Healy and Bigelow program was interrupted four to six times by the pitchman who would extol the virtues of nostrums from the Kickapoo Indian Medicine Company. A shill in the audience would buy a dollar bottle, sample it and proclaim himself cured, demanding another bottle. Floor salesmen -- usually performers doing double duty -- would carry only one or two bottles so that they could frequently holler, "All sold out, Doctor!" to feign frenzied buying, then rush to the stage for more provisions.

If this successful entertainment-interrupted-by-a-commercial format sounds familiar, it should; it has been adopted by radio and television broadcasters for their commercials!

These colorful characters had a slang of their own, using a "ballyhoo" (gimmick) to sell "slum" (liquid medicine), "grease" (salve), "chopped grass" (herbs), and "flea powder" (powdered herbs). They often associated with "pennyweighters" (diamond thieves), "moll buzzers" (purse snatchers) and "clock men" (watch thieves), and they employed "shills" (confederates) to "steer" (hustle) and "squeeze" (defraud) their "yokels" (suckers)!

High noon for the nostrum peddlers came on January 1st, 1907, with the passage into law of the 1906 Federal Pure Food and Drug Act, largely forced by the efforts of one tireless journalist, a reporter named Samuel Hopkins Adams. His scathing Collier's Weekly series, "The Great American Fraud," (Oct. 7, 1905-Sept. 22, 1906) exposed 264 swindling firms and hucksters.

After this expose', the federal government required these purveyors of potions to list the ingredients on their labels. It was not quackdom's finest hour, it was their final hour. The illegitimate empire began to crumble.

But patent medicines were far from extinct. Even after the passage of the 1906 Act, the Food and Drug Administration (FDA) gave food adulteration a higher enforcement priority than quack medicine. No jail sentences were imposed, and the small fines, typically $10-$50, were a minor business expense. Nostrum peddlers merely changed labels for appearances, and then claimed that their concoctions were endorsed by the FDA!

During the next few decades, automobiles, better roads, movie houses, radio and finally television, all provided alternative sources of entertainment to the old-time medicine shows. By the 1950s fewer than 10 road shows were left, and they were gone by the '60s when the last bottle of Hadacol was sold.

Hadacol was first concocted in the 1930s by Louisiana Senator Dudley J. "Coozin Dud" LeBlanc, a charismatic Cajun whose first batch of 140-proof vodka and Ever Clear alcohol with a dash of bitters and hydrochloric acid was mixed in a vat in his barn. By 1945 LeBlanc's Hadacol caravan rolled into towns, featuring entertainment by top entertainers, while blanketing several states with saturation advertising.

When the FDA put a stop to the Hadacol heyday, they asked LeBlanc, "What is Hadacol good for?" His reply was succinct: "It's good for about five million dollars a year to me!"

Few perpetrators really believed in their products; the overwhelming majority were then, as they are now, unconscionable charlatans. Legitimate physicians have historically derided this "gas pipe and wire" therapy, referring to Dr. Hercules Sanche's "Oxydonor" (1906-1911), made literally from gas pipe and wired to the body.

Government regulation of medical gadgetry began in earnest in 1938 with the passage of the Federal Food, Drug, and Cosmetic Act. Further restrictions have since been levied by the Medical Device Amendments of 1976 and the Safe Medical Devices Act of 1990.

But medical hucksterism continues to this day, with many individuals testifying to the miraculous healing they receive from devices, persons, icons, chemicals, and foods. Actor Steve McQueen believed coffee enemas would cure his cancer, while Peter Sellers engaged "psychic surgeons" in the Philippines. Both died of their maladies.

Americans are being bilked at least $25 billion a year by health scams. Gadgeteers often capitalize on high-tech fears like electromagnetic fields from power lines and cell phones.

Ads from a holistic magazine

A small amulet claims to balance, support, and protect you from "invisible energy drains," while a diode purports to hold you in electrical balance. Naturally, both are claimed to be used by doctors. For $19 plus shipping you can zap yourself electrically for instant pain relief. You can buy the same device -- a barbecue-grill spark igniter – for about $10 at Wal-Mart. For a mere $8 you can purchase a shower-curtain clip that assimilates your thought-sensitive energy field and stimulates your mind, soul and spirit. Send your photograph and $45 for a remote healing treatment--three treatments recommended.

As W.C. Fields philosophized in one of his movies, amending P.T. Barnum's famous quote: "There may be a sucker born every minute, but every ten minutes there's somebody born who'll take advantage of those suckers!"

Don't be fooled

So when is the treatment quackery? According to the FDA, if it's worthless or dangerous. For example, Davis and Kidder's shocking "Magneto Electric Machine" was promoted as a treatment for nervous disorders, but it's a good bet that the patient (victim?) was a lot more nervous after getting zapped! In any case, these devices don't live up to their claims. Let's look at the facts:

- No singular treatment (panacea or nostrum) is effective against a wide range of afflictions.
- No massager, external suction device, sauna, sweat device, cream, electrical or other gadget can take off weight or fat. Only diet or exercise can.
- Vibrators cannot cure arthritis, rheumatism, nervous disorders, heart conditions or other serious diseases.
- Breast enlargers don't work and can even cause the spreading of cancer cells if present.
- Home air purifiers, vacuum cleaners and negative ion generators cannot prevent or treat allergies, colds or other diseases.
- "Secret" treatments are fakes.
- Product endorsements and testimonials are worthless and often contrived.
- Pseudo-medical jargon like "detoxify," "purify" and "energize" are meaningless without measurements.

- Be wary of promotional hype like "100% guaranteed...amazing breakthrough...miraculous cure...natural and non-toxic."
- A potent cure will have some side effects; beware of claims that a product has none.
- Be suspicious of a treatment or product that is available from only one doctor, foundation, clinic or another country. If it really was a cure for a serious disease, it would be widely reported by the media and used by legitimate health care providers.
- Claims that a product is backed by scientific studies, but with no references, are suspect. Even if a real list is provided, studies may be fictitious, often out of date, irrelevant or poorly conducted.
- Accusations that a treatment or product is being suppressed by the medical profession, drug companies or the government are groundless. Why would physicians conspire to prevent useful treatments for their families, friends and clients?

If you have a question about a medical device, treatment or compound, contact your nearest FDA office. If you wish to report a suspect device or remedy, send complete information to the Office of Compliance, Food and Drug Administration, 10903 New Hampshire Ave., Rockville, MD 20993-0002; (301) 796-3100.

COLLECTIBLE DEVICES
Most vintage contrivances fall into one of several categories:
- Passive devices (bracelets, anklets, collars, belts, rollers, plasters, amulets)
- Batteries (Galvanic electrodes)
- Faradic batteries (vibrating-contact spark coils)
- Induction coils ("horse collars")

- Magnetos (hand-cranked electromagnetic generators)
- Electrostatic generators (Wimshurst machines with leads)
- Violet ray generators (glass electrodes that glow blue from high-voltage-ionized nitrogen gas)
- Vacuum-tube radio-frequency devices
- Magnets
- Radioactive substances
- Diagnostic contraptions

Such contraptions of questionable therapeutic value often glow, blink, buzz, click, or shock in an attempt to impress the patient. Common on the collector's market are the wood-encased Faradic batteries from roughly 1880-1910, and the violet ray devices of the 1920s and 30s. Modern versions are still being manufactured and sold through alternative medical catalogs.

Quack medical collections are few and far between. There is no organized collecting society, but informational exchange is growing on the Internet. Many copycat devices are still on the market and, just as with patent medicines, one manufacturer might private-label products for a variety of companies, or they may simply be copied by independent promoters.

The most productive sources of quack medical devices for collectors, in descending order, are: eBay, antique radio and amateur radio swap meets and magazines, antique shops, flea markets, yard sales, estate sales, and auctions.

GLOSSARY OF TERMS

Electrode: The electrical attachment to the patient: a glass tube, metal prod, cylinder, plate, or wet cotton.

Faradic battery/medical battery: An electro-shock device utilizing a battery-powered induction coil.

Faradic current: The pulsating direct current produced by an induction coil.

Galvanic current: The direct current produced by a cell or battery.

Induction coil: A battery powered, high-voltage-output transformer utilizing a spark-contact interrupter in its primary winding to produce pulsating (Faradic) current.

CATALOGING AND VALUATION

As with other antiques, value is what the traffic will bear, and market prices vary enormously with condition, completeness, rarity, demand and the seller's knowledge. The flea market axiom: If you don't know what it is, it's $25; if it's big, it's $100.

The emergence of eBay and televised antique and auction programs have had a profound impact on the resale market. Violet ray devices and Faradic batteries which were formerly $25 are now bringing $50-$100 or more. But bargains are still out there.

Faradic batteries were in wide distribution from the 1880s to 1920s, consisting of one or two carbon/zinc "A" size dry cells which powered a spark coil. The low-voltage direct current from the cells was transformed into pulsating DC by a spark-gap interrupter (vibrating contacts) at the end of the large, adjustable coil.

Virtually all of these devices were in oak boxes with hinged lids. Wires were attached to two tubular metal electrodes which, in turn, were applied to the patient (victim?) who would feel anywhere from a mild tingle to a whopping shock depending upon how the interrupter (spark gap) was set, where the electrodes were applied, the condition of the batteries, and how sweaty the patient was by the time he got the treatment.

Dimensions listed below are width, height, and depth in inches. Years of manufacture are approximate.

PRODUCT LIST (**NOTE:** Descriptions of therapeutic benefits are claims made by the manufacturer, not the author!)

Passive Devices

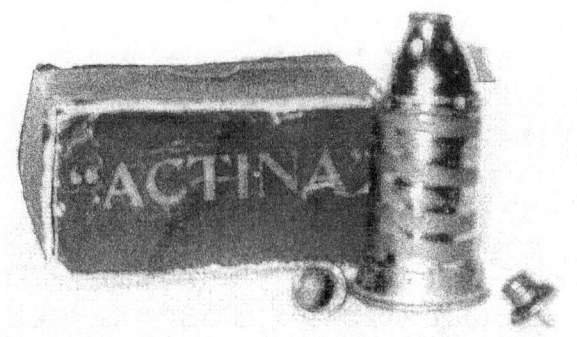

Actina (1894, William C. Wilson); 3" cylindrical metal inhaler/applicator, flared end for eye, swaged end for nose.

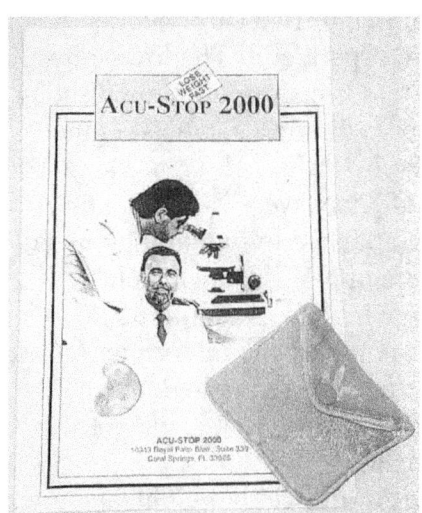

Acu-Stop 2000 weight reducer; rubber ear insert is massaged.

Addison's Galvanic Electric Belt (1915, $2.50, Electric Appliance Company) For rheumatism, liver, kidneys, paralysis, poor circulation, stomach, lame back and all nervous diseases.

Adrenoray (1930; William J.A. Bailey) Belt with five discs allegedly containing radium for adrenal therapy.

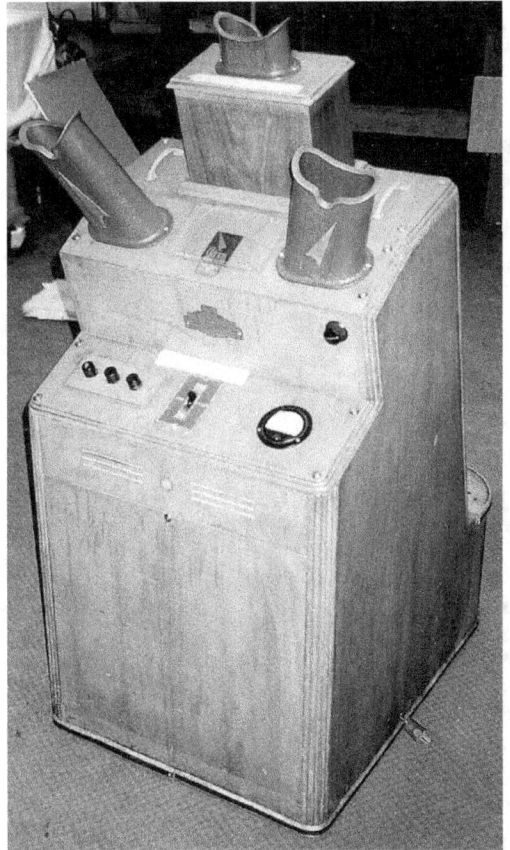

Adrian shoe-fitting fluoroscope Banned in 1970s because of dangerous X-radiation

Aerobic Eye exerciser.

Arden Copper bracelet.
Artificial Ear Drum Tiny, insertable ear trumpet.
Babylon's Zone Therapy Roller (1950s)
Baldness Cap (French, 1940s) Pulsating vacuum stimulates the scalp to encourage hair growth.

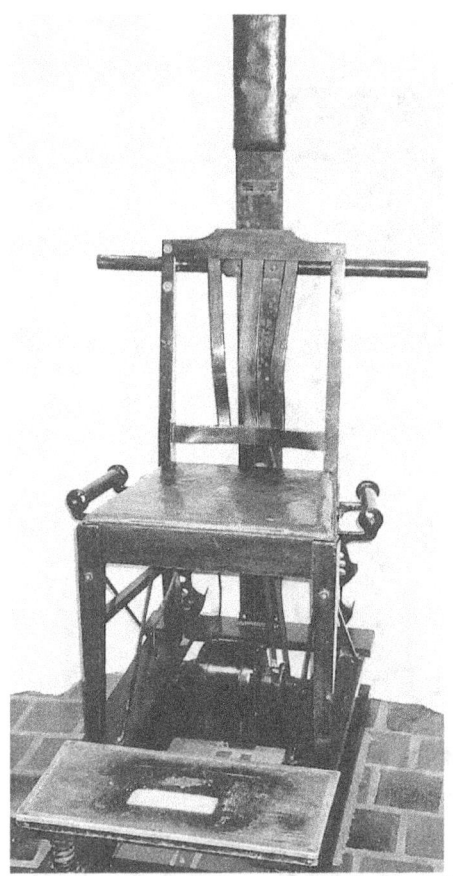

Battle Creek Vibratory Chair (Dr, Kellogg, 1900) Violent vibration stimulates intestinal peristalsis, cures headaches and back pain, and increases "healthy" oxygen supply to the body.

Bleeding cups (glass, 1830-1850)

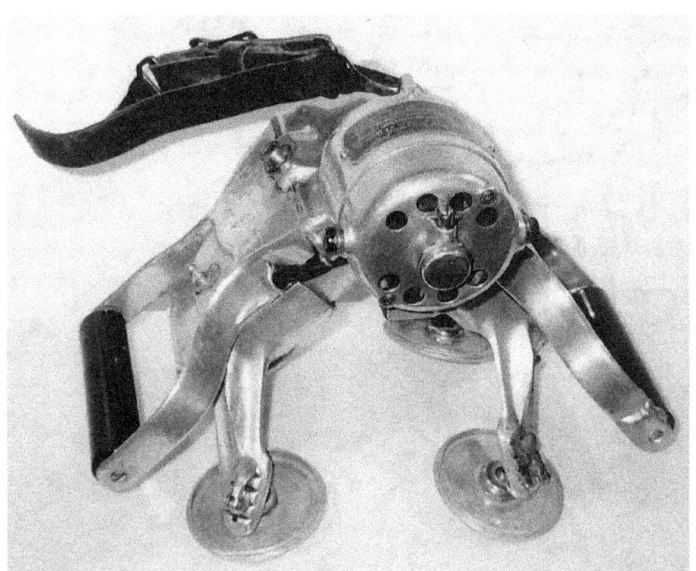

Blud Rub Vibrator

Breast exerciser/enlarger (1976) Foot pump connected by hoses to two suction cups (Ouch!).
Cartilage contraption (1905-1915, Charles S. Clark, Thomas Adkin) Cast iron bar, pulleys, ropes, straps, stirrups to increase height.

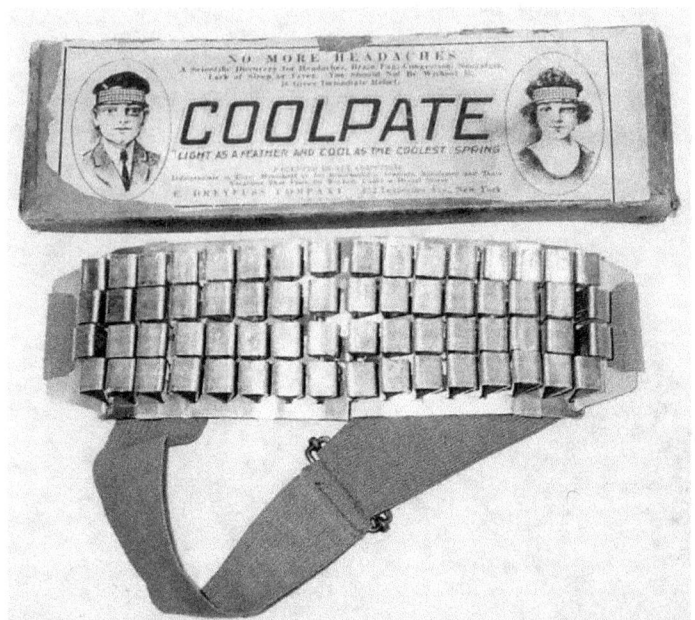

Coolpate (1902) Metal band wrapped across the forehead to alleviate headaches.

Copper ("electric") bracelet (1950s-90s) Primarily hawked as arthritis cure.

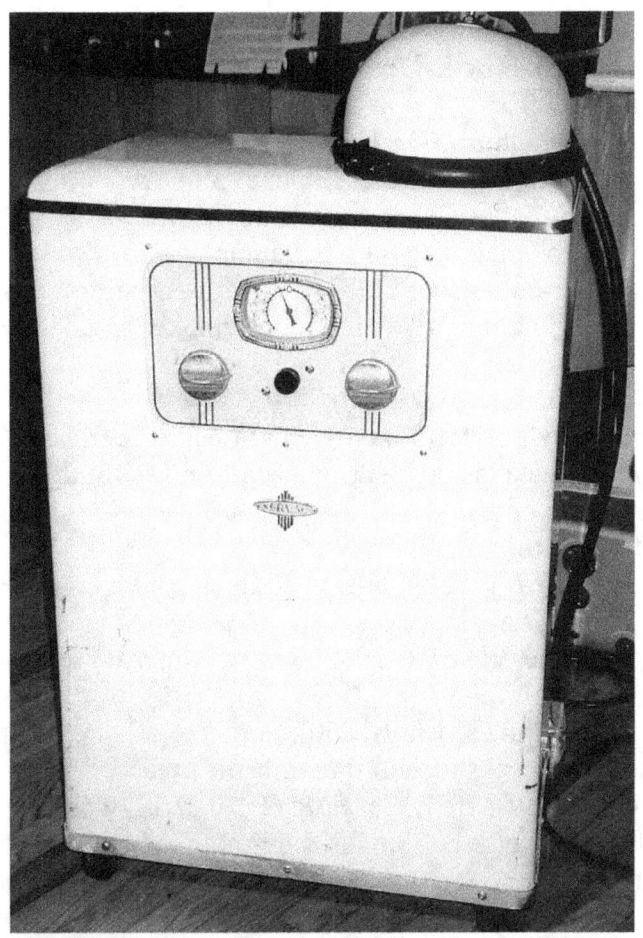

Crosley Xervac (Crosley Radio Corp.) Hair growing machine, consisting of a skull cap, suction hose, and a white console with three knobs and a gauge.

Dr. Coutant's Nasal Douche (1910-12, George E. Coutant) Nickel-plated 3x1/2 tube, one ended swaged, other rounded; alternatively a glass tube with side bowl, closed at one end, other end open and offset; for treatment of deafness.

Electric ring (Sears) Polished grey metal ($.50) or gold-plated grey metal ($.95) for rheumatism.

Electro-Chemical Ring (1892-1915, W.G. Brownson) Iron finger ring, inner stamp "E-C"; cures diseases caused by acid in the blood.

Electro-Magnetic Chain (Dr. Raphael)

Electropoise (1893, Dr. Hercules Sanche) 5 ounce, hollow, sealed, metal cylinder, attached to stranded, uninsulated wire, connected to small disc on wrist/ankle band..

Fedelerizer Food-enhancing blood vitalizer consisting of a lidded glass jar containing two electrodes, hooked to an AC cord.

Glasseptic nebulizer

Heidelberg Electric Belt (Sears, 1880s) Leather, canvas and satin; multiple cells and electrodes within; for youthful vigor and multiple cures.

Hollywood Vita-Rol

Ideal Sight Restorer (1880s) U-shaped device with cups on each end to press against eyes.

Isotron Figuretone set 1910-1917 Rubber water bottle with rectal enema syringe

Lancet (bleeding knives, 1830-1850).

Life Awakener Awl for penetrating arthritic areas.

J.B.L. ("Joy-Beauty-Life") Cascade (1910-1917, Charles A. Tyrell) Rubber water bottle with side-mounted rectal enema syringe.

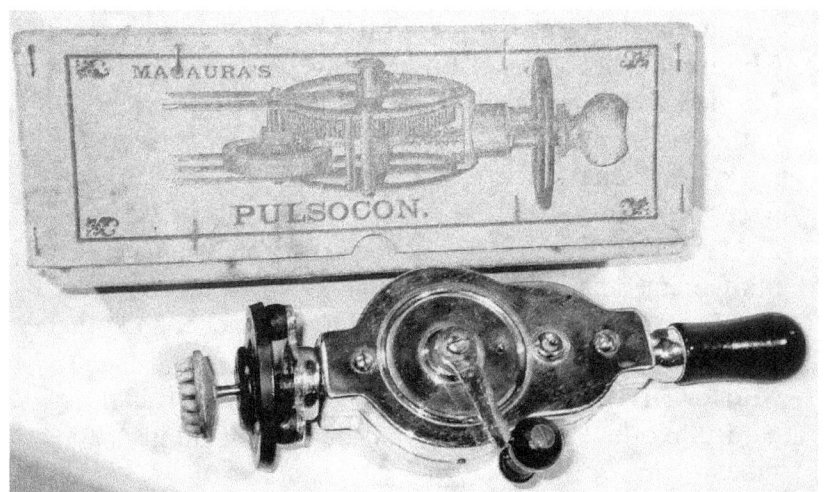

Macaura Pulsator (1910-1915, "Pulsocon," "Cirkulon." Gerald Macaura) Hand-cranked, stomping vibrator for curing pain and improving blood circulation.

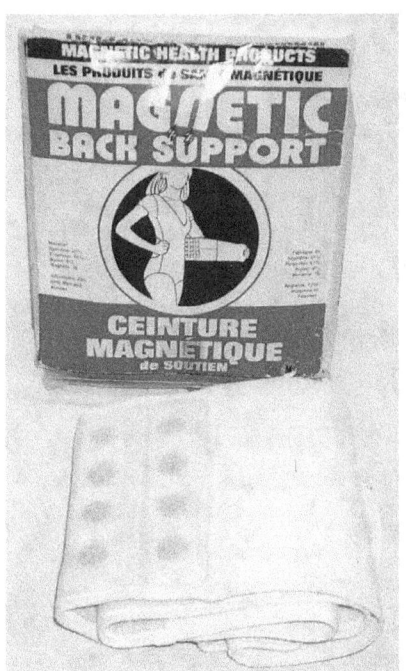

Magnetic Products magnetic back support

Magnetic-Ray Belt "Horse Collar."

Magnetic shield (Dr. C.J. Thacher)

Magic Flesh Builder/Cupper (Sears, $.50) Squeeze-bulb with suction cup; to remove wrinkles and smooth bust, neck, arms, cheeks.

Memory Band (1912, $17.50 per dozen) Japanese copy of the 1902 Coolpate; rubber-banded, flexible head strap of alloy metal squares; measures 6.4"x2.75"; cures fatigue, nasal bleeding, apoplexy, neuralgia, toothache, and other illnesses due to blood stagnation.

Morley Invisible Ear-Phone (1911-1913) Artificial eardrum; oiled silk disk, waxed silk thread and insertion tube.

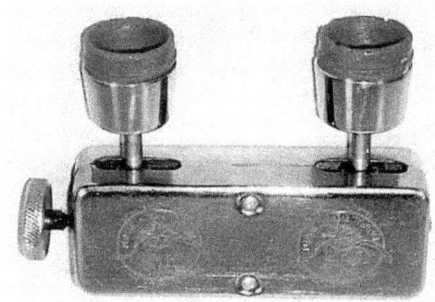

Natural Eye Normalizer (1930s, $30) to restore 20/20 vision; small, nickel-plated rectangular box with two protruding, rubber-cupped cylinders to apply twirling pressure to the eyeballs; side knob adjusts spacing.

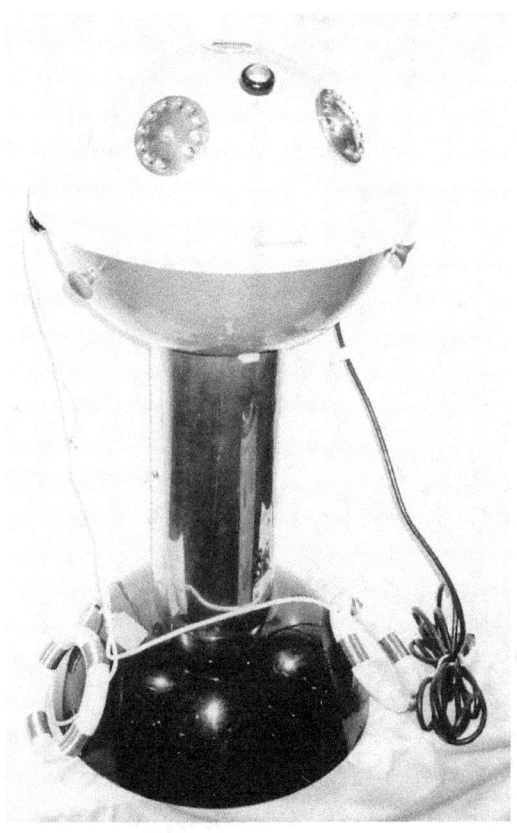

Nemectron (1950s) Body toner; chrome-plated pedestal with hemispherical base and spherical top; two ear rings for regenerating brain cells.

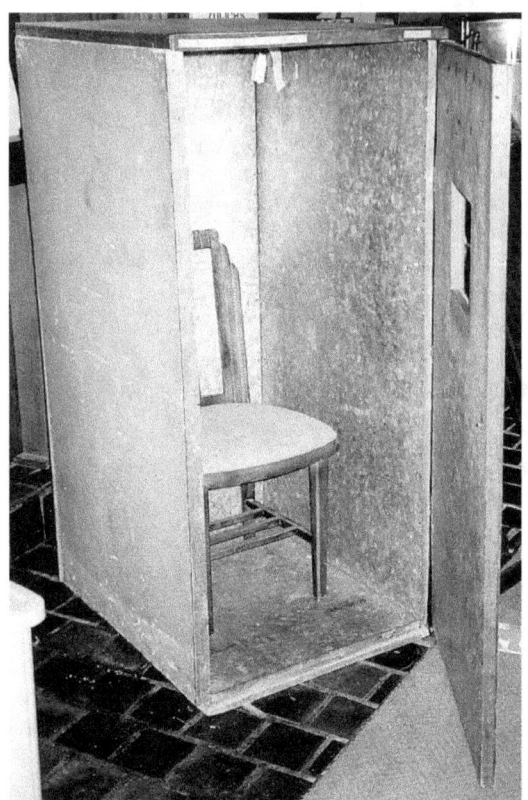

Orgone Energy Accumulator (1938-1950; Dr. Wilhelm
Reich) Sheet-metal-lined wood enclosure containing a chair
and a funnel-shaped breathing mask.

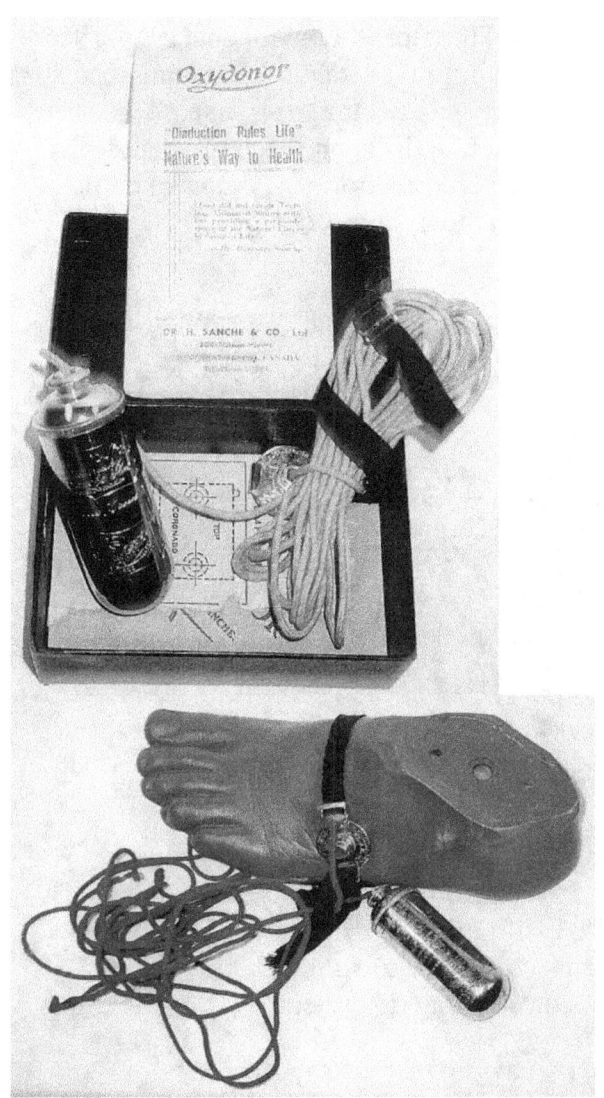

Oxydonor (1895-1916, Dr. Hercules Sanche) and demonstration mockup. Short metal cylinder (1.25" x 3.25") containing carbon rod placed in water, attached to stranded, uninsulated wire connected to a small disc. Attachments included the Animator, Novora, Binora, and Vocorbis.

Oxybon (Competitive imitator of Oxydonor) (1910-1916, Dr. Filloon, Ben A. Hallgren) Metal tube containing sulfur, ash and carbon, end caps connected to stranded, uninsulated wires attach to disks on wrist/ankle garters.
Oxygenator (Competitive imitator of Oxydonor; named changed later to Oxypathor).

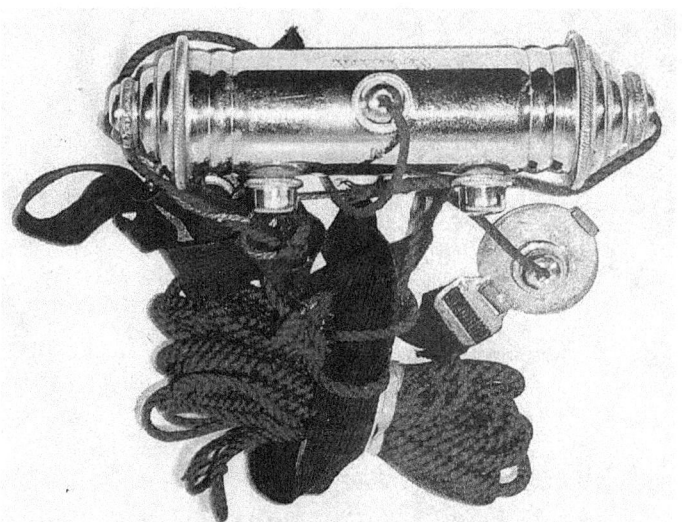

Oxygenor-King (Competitive imitator of Oxydonor) (1910-1915, $25, Woodford M. Davis) Nickel-plated copper tube filled with mixture of sulfur, sand and charcoal; end caps connected to stranded, bare wires attached to disks on wrist/ankle garters.

Oxypathor (1910-1915, $25-$35, Elvard L. Moses) Competitive imitator of Oxydonor. Nickel-plated copper tube filled with a black powder, capped at both ends, connected by stranded, bare wire to metal disks on two elastic wrist/ankle garters.
Oxtytonor Competitive imitator of Oxydonor.

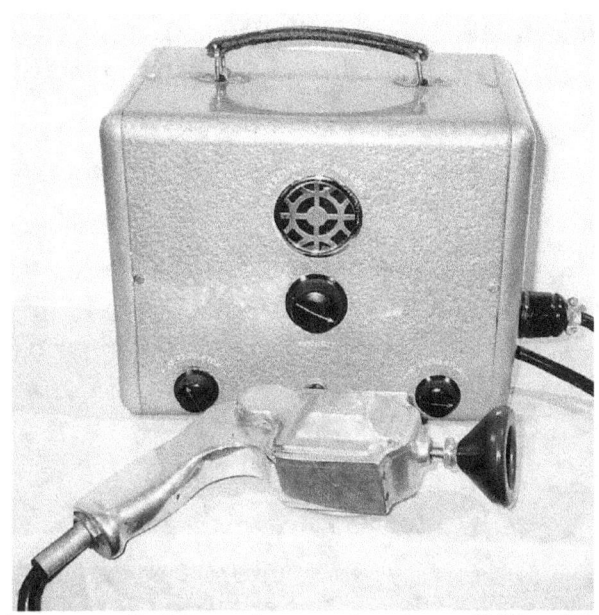

Percuss-O-Motor heart stimulator (10" x 8" x 7")

Perkins' Tractors (1795, Dr. Elisha Perkins) Two three-inch, pointed, brass and iron rods used to massage.

Pol-izer (1957) Glass tube containing mercury to "pol-ize" oxygen water for purification and to sweeten bad wine.

Phrenology Machine (1905) Metal head gear with adjustable prods to measure bumps on the head.

Princess Bust Developer (Sears, $1.50)) Nickel and aluminum syringe pump with either 3-1/2" or 5" cup.

Professor Wilson's Magneto-Conservative Insoles (See Magneto-Conservative Insoles).

Pulvermacher's Electro-Galvanic Chain (1890s)

Rectal dilator Probe for inserting into rectum to relieve hemorrhoids.

Res-Q-Air (1960s) Plastic bellows emergency respirator with mouthpiece.

Richardson's Magneto-Galvanic Battery (1880s) Round disk with magnets worn as an amulet to cure wide variety of diseases.

Sanden electric belt (1905-1914, A.T. Sanden).
Sauna suits (1970s-80s) Rubber-like body wraps promoted
to reduce weight.

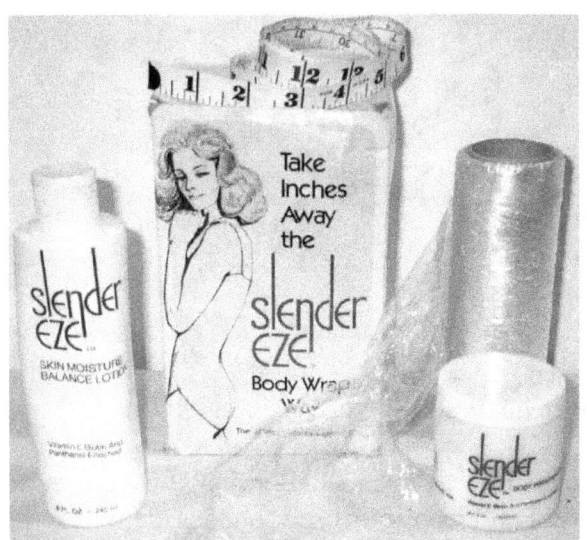

Slender Eze Body Wrap for weight reduction

Slendro Ring Roller (MacLevy, 1957, $895) Motor-
driven massager in six-foot framework weighing 650
pounds; guarantees to roll off 1-3 inches in ten applications.

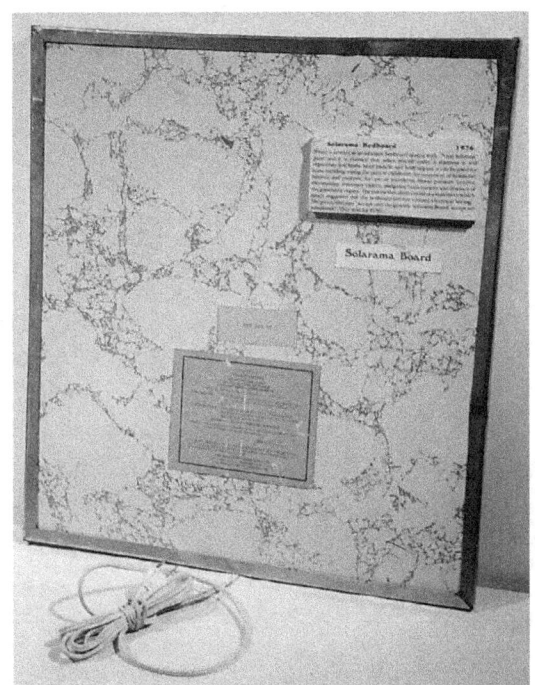

Solarama Board

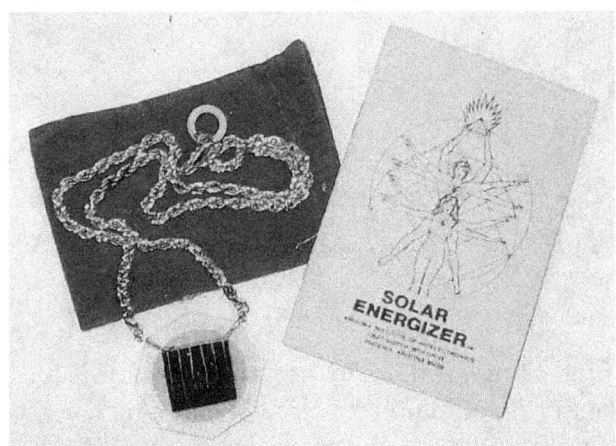

Solar Energizer

Sonus Film-O-Sonic Machine Plays "silent" recorded music for therapeutic effect.

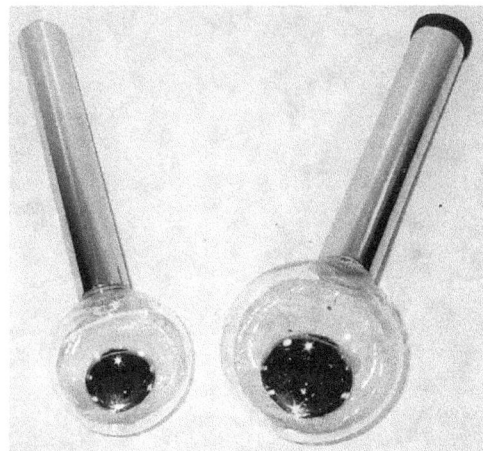

Therapeutic Wands

Thermapax Magnetic Wave Helmet Domed metal helmet.

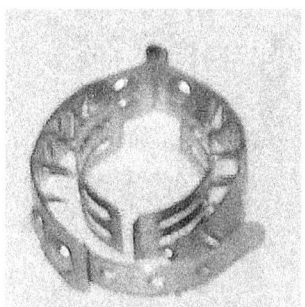

Timely Warning Ring (1905) This erection deflator is a hinged aluminum ring containing pointed teeth which close around penis to discourage nocturnal erection (Ouch!)

Vibrating belts (1960s-70s) Motor-driven belts promoted to reduce weight.

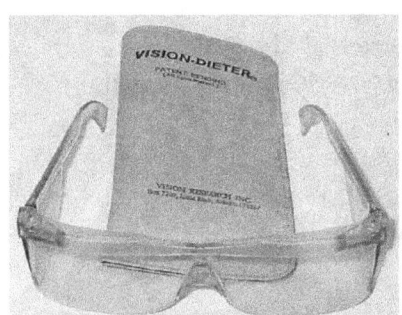

Vision-Dieter Plastic eyeglasses with one blue and one brown lens, curbs appetite.

Vitalizer Metal cylinder containing powdered iron oxide, immersed in ice water.

Vital Power Vacuum Massager Strapped to the body, this device was "the perfect organ developing appliance."

Vrilium Tube (1948; George Erickson and Robert Nelson) Two-inch brass tube, 1/2"D., contains glass tube of barium chloride attached to clothing by safety pin.

Wahl Powersage Vibrator massager

Way Artificial Ear Drum (1913, George P. Way) Two rubber, horn-shaped ear canal inserts.

White Cross Electric Vibrator Chair (Lindstrom, Smith Co.) No. 27 Model B massager with accessories, black leatherette case with nickel-plated corner protectors, 14"x10.5"x4.5".

Wilson Ear-Drum (1913) Two rubber ear canal inserts; originally included forceps and inserters.

Zerret Applicator (1948; William R. Ferguson) Dumbbell of blue and white plastic globes containing plastic tubes of water.

Batteries

Body Battery

Dr. Dye's Voltaic Belt (1890s, Pulvermacher) "Electric" belt.

Dr. John Wilson Gibbs Electricura Shoes to cure rheumatism; "A positive battery in the heel of one and a negative battery in the other."

Dr. Owens' Body Battery Electro-galvanic belt, $6 in 1887, to cure nervous disorders and many diseases.

Dr. Scott's Electric Corset and Belt $1-$3 in 1905.

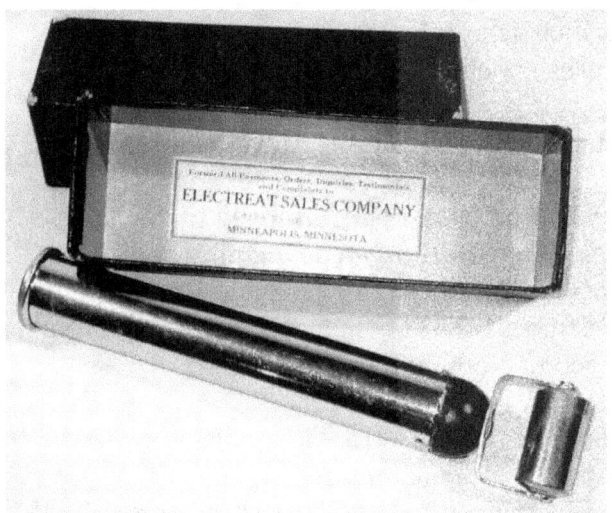

Electreat apparatus (1928-1938) Cylinder with roller on end, containing two D cells; accessories included sponge, scalp brush, and palm-massage pad; intended for physical therapy, pain relief, lithesome busts, and hair growth.

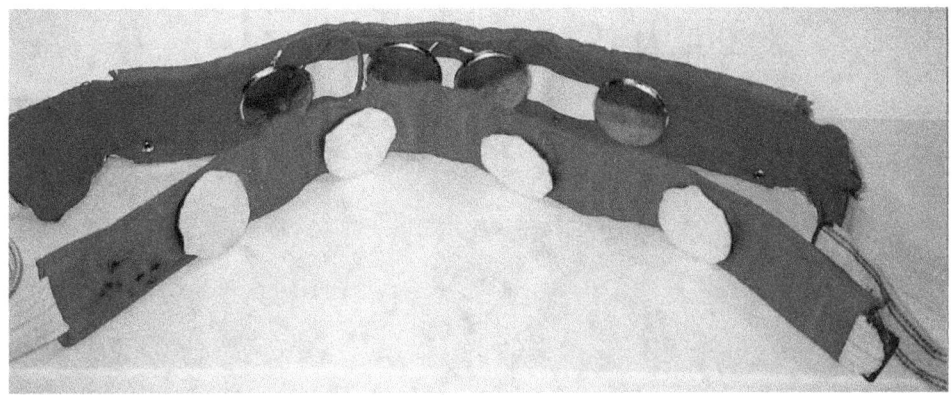

Electric belt

Electric Battery Plasters Apply to region of back and kidney pain.
Electric Body Battery/Mioxrl (1891-1915, Electric Appliance Company) Belt of red and yellow cotton strips containing copper and zinc plates separated by blotting paper (to be dipped in sulfuric acid or vinegar); for strengthening sexual organs (male and female versions) as well as curing many diseases.
Electric Slippers
Electric Truss
Electricura Shoes (see Dr. John Wilson Gibbs)
Morse Electric Belt Claimed to cure all diseases..
Nap-A-Night device Russian sleep machine in black leatherette case, hinged top, white panel with control and D cell holder, electric cord to goggles and neck piece.
Voltaic belt (1890)

Violet Ray Devices

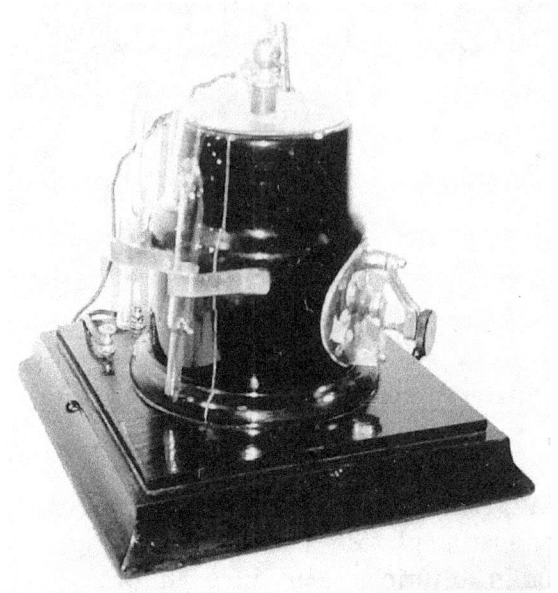

Early violet ray device (1895; 10" x 10" x10")

Challenge Ray (1927, $7.95, Sears, Roebuck) Violet ray device in black leatherette carrying case, 3 glass electrodes.

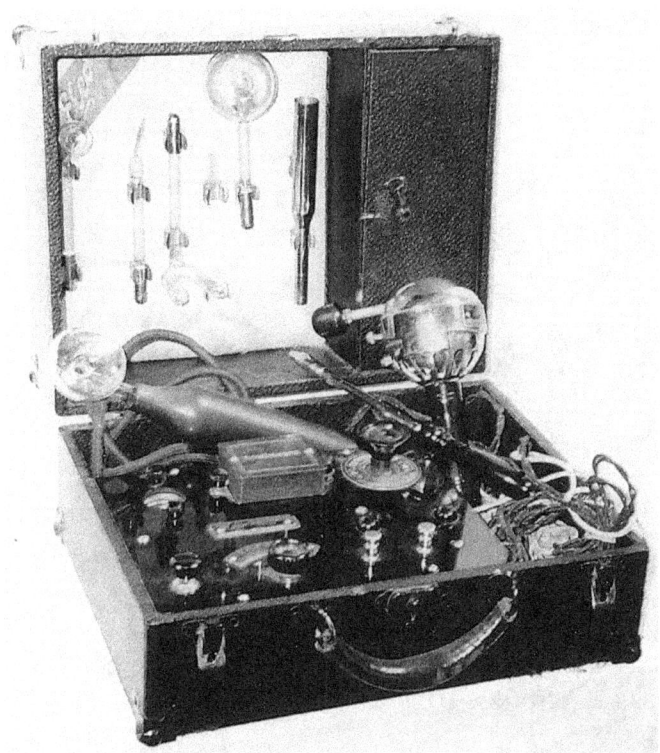

Elco (Lindstrom & Co.) Combination Health Generator
No. 12 (1927) Violet ray generator, 6 glass electrodes,
ozone mask, vibrator massager, miscellaneous probes and
accessories, black-leatherette case.

Elco (Lindstrom & CO.) Electric Health Generator No. 9
(1926); violet ray generator, 2 glass electrodes, vibrator
massager, miscellaneous probes and accessories, black
leatherette case.
Elco (Lindstrom & Co.) Electric Health Generator No. 38
(1927) High frequency violet ray apparatus, 5 glass and 1
metal electrode, ozone mask, black leatherette case,
11.5"x8.75"x5.5".
Elco (Lindstrom & Co.) violet ray induction coil only,
black case, 10"x6"x3".

Energex Violet Ray (1927, $12.75, Sears, Roebuck) Black leatherette case, 5 glass electrodes.

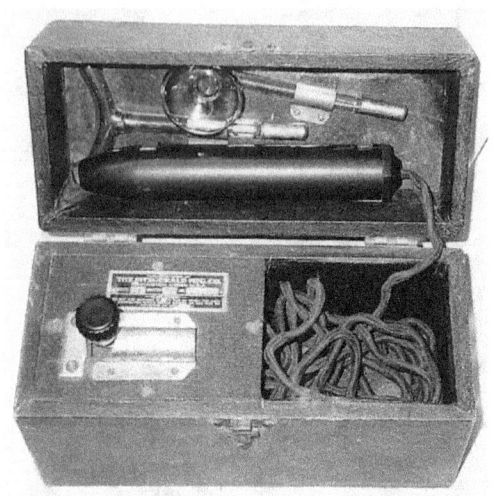

Fitzgerald violet ray generator (1925) Black leatherette case, 2 glass electrodes, 10.5"x4.5"x7.25".

Halliwell-Shelton Violet Ray 3 glass electrodes, black leatherette case, 13"x8.75"x3.25".

Marvel No. A1 violet ray generator (1924) Violet ray device, basic; one general-purpose glass electrode.

Marvel, Super No. 3 violet ray generator (1926) 3 glass electrodes, black leatherette case, 13.25"x9"x3.5".

Marvel Special No. 5/5B violet ray generator, 5 electrodes.

Marvel Ozone No. 7 Violet ray generator, 5 electrodes, bottle of inhalant.

Master violet ray generator (various models) Glass electrodes, wand, induction coil, in black leatherette case,

Ozone Generator Set (1927, $18.75, Sears, Roebuck) Violet ray device in black leatherette case, several glass electrodes, inhaler, inhalant.

RenuLife Generator model 2-120 (1919) Violet ray apparatus, 2 glass electrodes, ivory-wood panel, black leatherette case, 11.5"x9"x4".

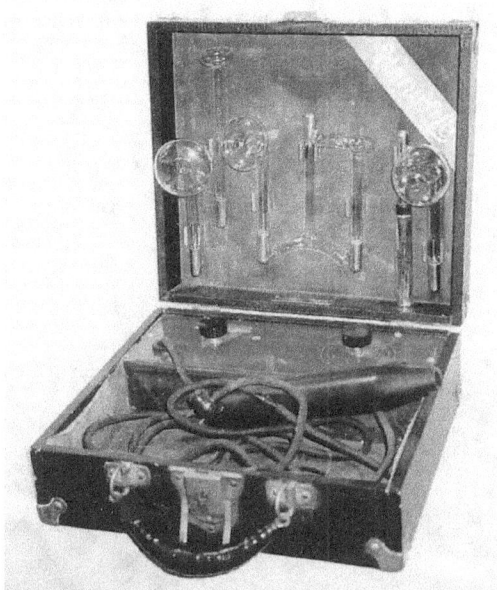

RenuLife violet ray generator, model M

RenuLife Violet Ray Generator, Model K 5 glass electrodes, cherry control panel, black leatherette carrying case.
RenuLife Violet Ray Generator, Model R (1922) 11 glass electrodes, ozone generator, cherry control panel, black leatherette case with nickel-plated hardware, lock latch and corner protectors, 15"x10.5"x5.5".
Shelton White Cross and White Cross violet ray generator.
Tucker's violet ray device
Violet ray generator (generic) Green leatherette case, 3 glass electrodes, 12"x6.5"x3".

Violetta, Baby, Type A Violet ray set (1924); leatherette case, 10x3x5-1/2; one general-purpose glass electrode.
Violetta Multifrex Violet Ray Apparatus, Type B Leatherette case, three-way function switch, one general purpose glass electrode.
Violetta Outfit, No. 1 Violet ray set; leatherette case, one general-purpose glass electrode.
Violetta Outfit, No. 3 Violet ray set, leatherette case; with comb rake, eye, throat, and metal electrodes.
Violetta De Luxe Outfit, No. 10 Mahogany or white enamel box, white marble top panel; 6"x5"x4.5"; one general purpose, glass electrode.

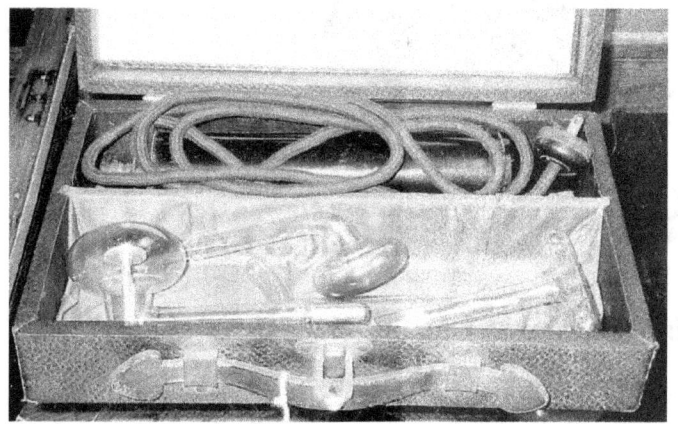

Violetta violet ray device Vi-Rex Electric Company, Chicago, IL (12.5" x 7.5" x 3")

Electroshock therapy

Advance Electric shock machine.

Aloe Lightning Electro-Therapeutic Outfit Black leatherette briefcase, white marble top panel, 0-1000 mA. meter, adjustable spark gap, two rotary switches (4 and 20 position) with exposed stud contacts, approximately a dozen glass and metal electrodes and applicators mounted in hinged lid.

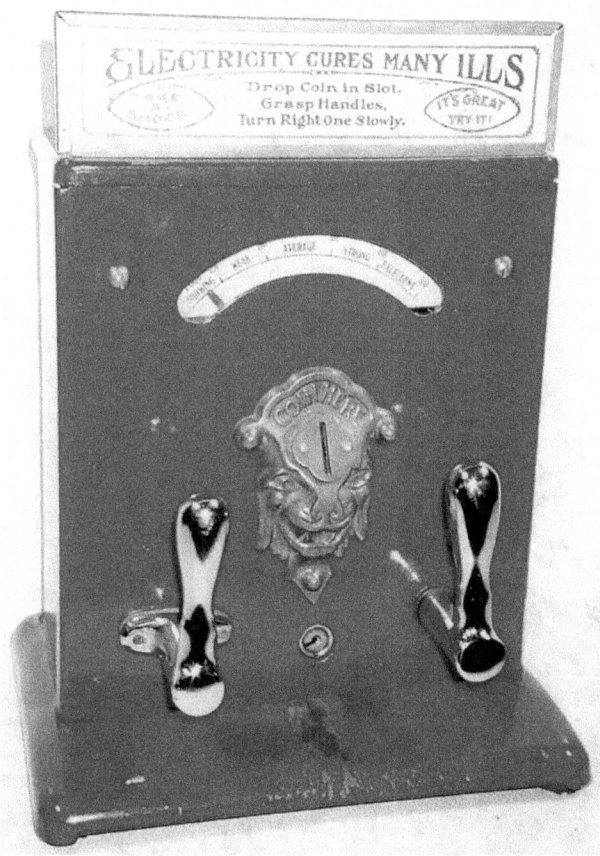

Arcade Shock Therapy coin operated (8" x 7" x 10")

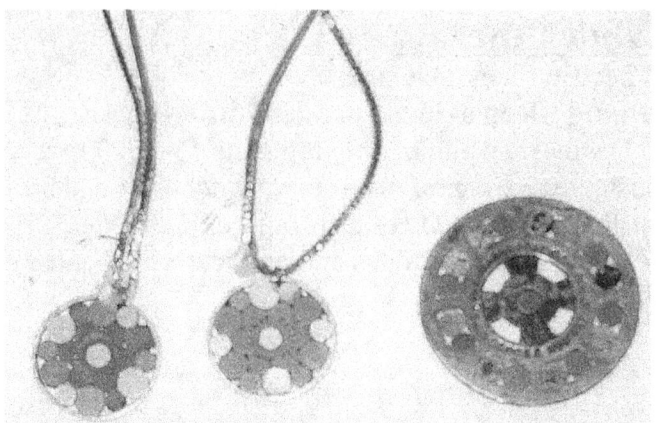

Boyd's Galvanic Battery (1878) A round amulet ostensibly worn to produce a constant, gentle flow of invigorating electricity into the body.

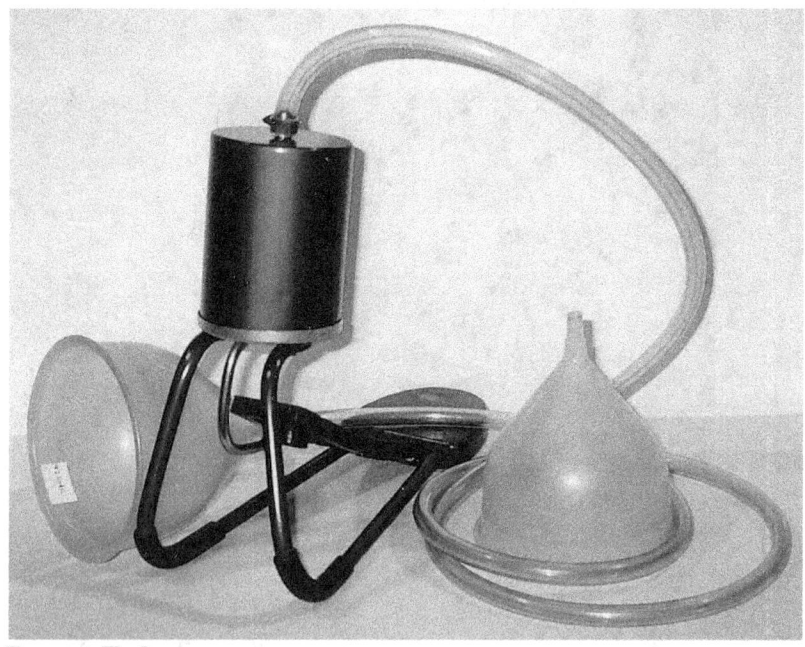

Breast Enlarger

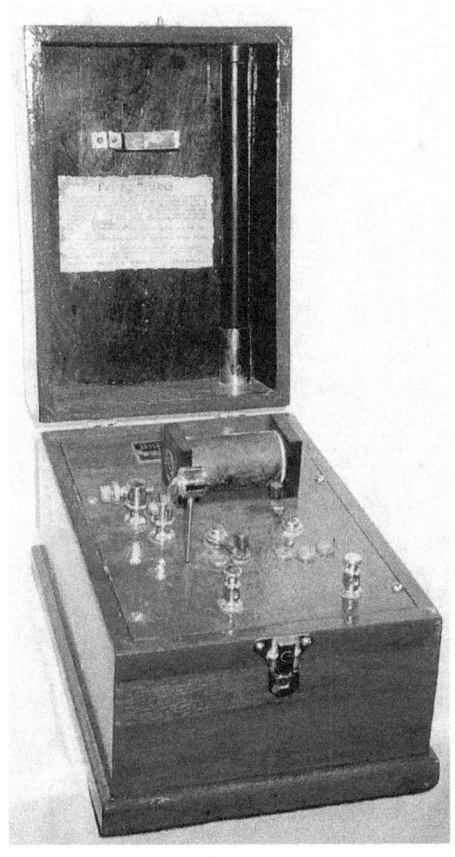

Bristow Coil (McIntosh Battery and Optical Company; 8" x 8" x 11.5")

Bunnel medical battery (wood case)
Chiropra Therapeutic Comb (1950s; Dr. Theodore Schwartz, Mannheim Germany).

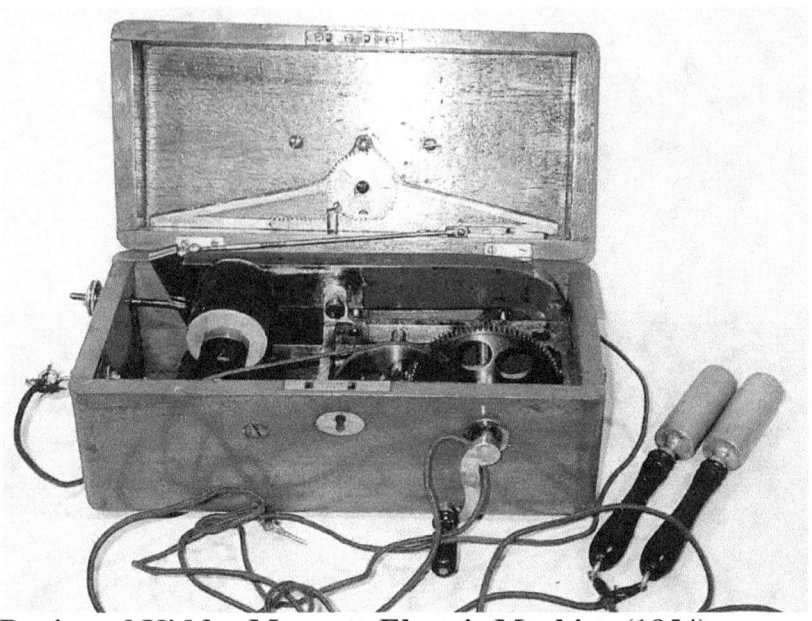

Davis and Kidder Magneto Electric Machine (1854), imprinted "W.H. Burnap Street, New York."

D'Arsonval's Thermo-Faradic machine (1909) Oak paneled cabinet, brass ball electrodes on top, 30" x 23" x 41".

Dr. Jerome Kidder's Celebrated Electro Magnetic machine.

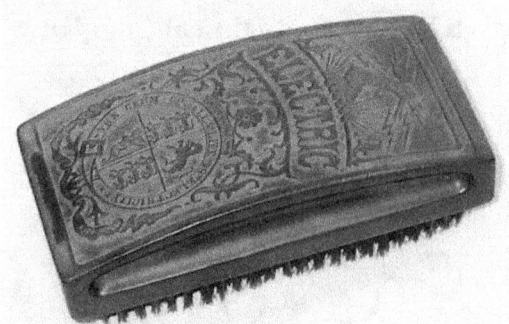

Dr. Scott's Electric Hair Brush (1905; three sizes) Internal magneto pumped by thumb pressure.

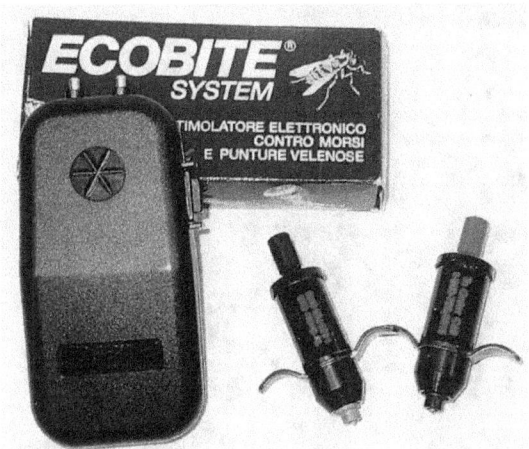

Ecobite electric stimulator

Electricity is Life (1920s-30s) Penny-operated arcade shock machine; 0-500 gauge, two metal knobs for gripping.
Electrification machine (1875) Magneto, electrodes, wood box.
Electro-Magnetic Hair Brush and Comb (1900, Actina Appliance Co.).
Electro medical machine Oak box, Sears Roebuck catalog item.

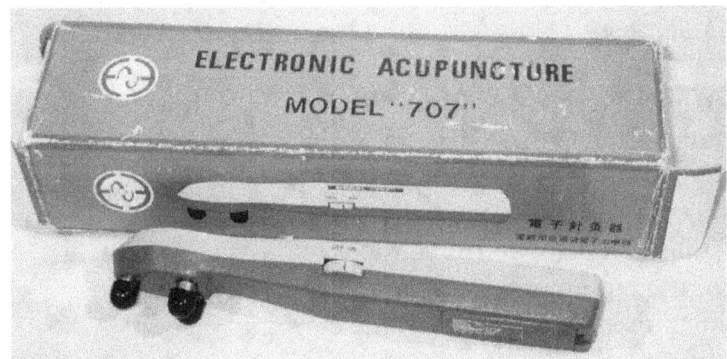

Electronic Acupuncture model 707

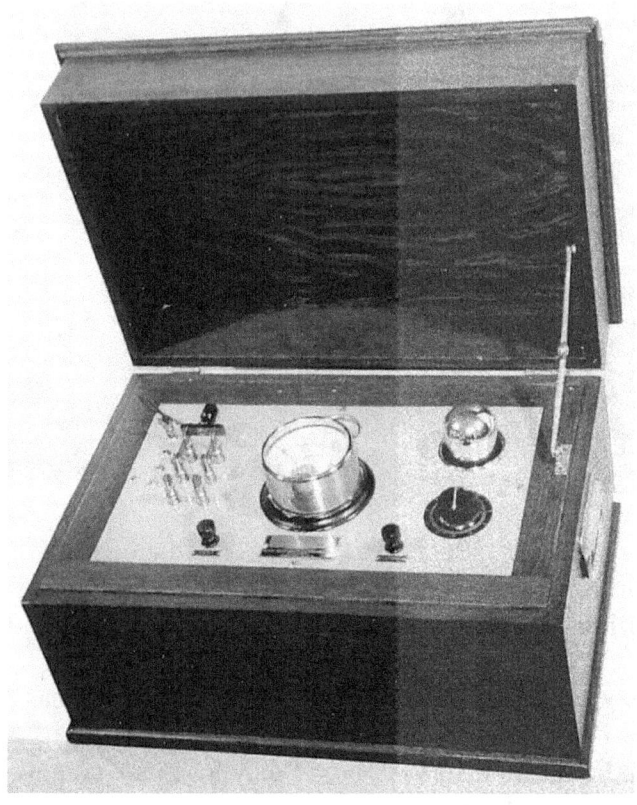

Electroshock device in hinged-lid cabinet (Unidentified manufacturer)

Electro Sine Galvanic Model 200 (L.L. Roby Manufacturing Corp. Tiffin, OH) suitcase contains a switch, pilot lights, 0-25 DC mA meter, and several knobs to adjust current type, intensity and frequency; outlets for plugging in foot switch, electrodes, cloth pads and metal strips; used to produce surged, pulsating or continuous faradic pulses as well as galvanic current.

Faradic Battery (various) Induction coil apparatus in oak wood box, hinged lid, cylindrical metal electrodes; nickel-plated grounding plate mounted inside lid.

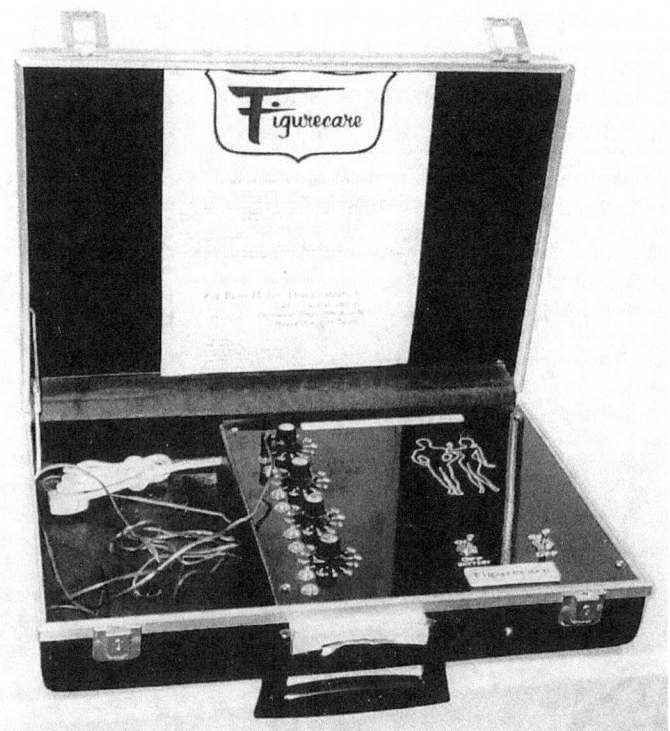

Figurecare

Fitness Machine Model EE-400/ Ultratonic (1990s) briefcase electric muscle stimulator (EMS) induces electric currents into the body to produce involuntary contractions.

Frank S. Betz faradic battery Black leatherette carrying case containing induction coil on green panel; two cylindrical metal electrodes connected by red and green wires to pin jacks.

Galvanic device (no name) Cherry box with hinged lid houses battery and electrodes, rheostat on lid, Bakelite binding posts on side, 7" x 3"x 1.75".

Galvanic Rejuvenating machine (1872) Cherry wood box.

Gem Battery (1906, Sears, Roebuck) Induction coil in walnut box; lower compartment holds nickel-plated dry-cell cylinder; upper compartment holds 2 metal electrodes, 2 wood handles, 1 sponge electrode, 2 cords, 1 nickel-plated foot plate.

Magneto box (1900) Wooden box, hinged top lid, front crank, internal magneto with gear train connected by two wires to hand-held electrodes.

Magneto-Electric machine (1854) Burled walnut box, brass works.

Mechanical Heart electro-treatment device (1928).

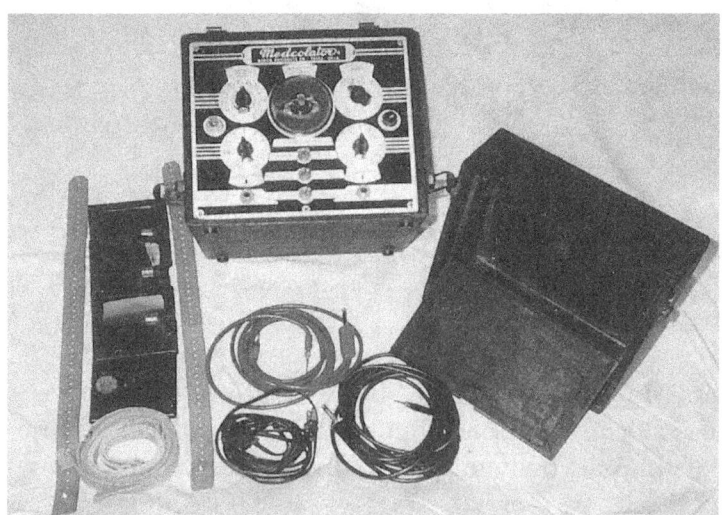

Medcolator 50B (1950s-1980s) Electro shock device with 4 paddles (4"x4"), 2 wrist and leg straps, 2 body straps, 2 signal leads, 1 type 1619 vacuum tube; internal speaker makes a sound during use.

Medicine Man homeopathic shock device (1880) Oak wooden box.

Medical Battery (1927, $12.45, Sears, Roebuck) Induction coil in oak box, 2 dry cells, pole-reversing switch, nickel-plated hardware, slide-adjustable vibrator with scale, hair brush, nickel-plated foot plate, 2 hand electrodes, 2 wooden handles, 2 sponge electrodes, 2 cords, 1 metallic scourge.

Medical Battery (1906, Sears, Roebuck) Induction coil in oak box, 3 dry cells, pole-reversing switch, nickel-plated hardware, 3-1/4" carbon rheostat, hair brush, nickel-plated foot plate, 2 hand electrodes, 2 wood handles, 2 sponge electrodes, 2 cords, 1 metallic scourge.

Medical Battery (1927, Sears, Roebuck) 3 models: triple, double and single dry cell; induction coil device in black leatherette case, two cords, two wooden handles, two metal handles, two sponge electrodes, one nickel-plated foot plate.

Otto Fleming faradic battery (1898) Oak box, hinged lid, nickel-plated hardware, induction coil, 2 metal electrodes.

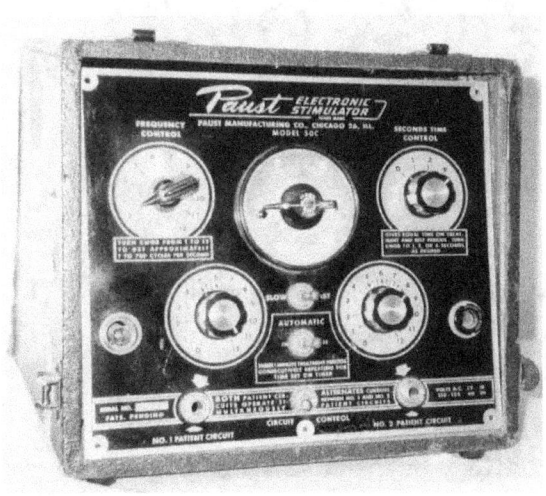

Paust Electronic Stimulator; model 50C (1950)

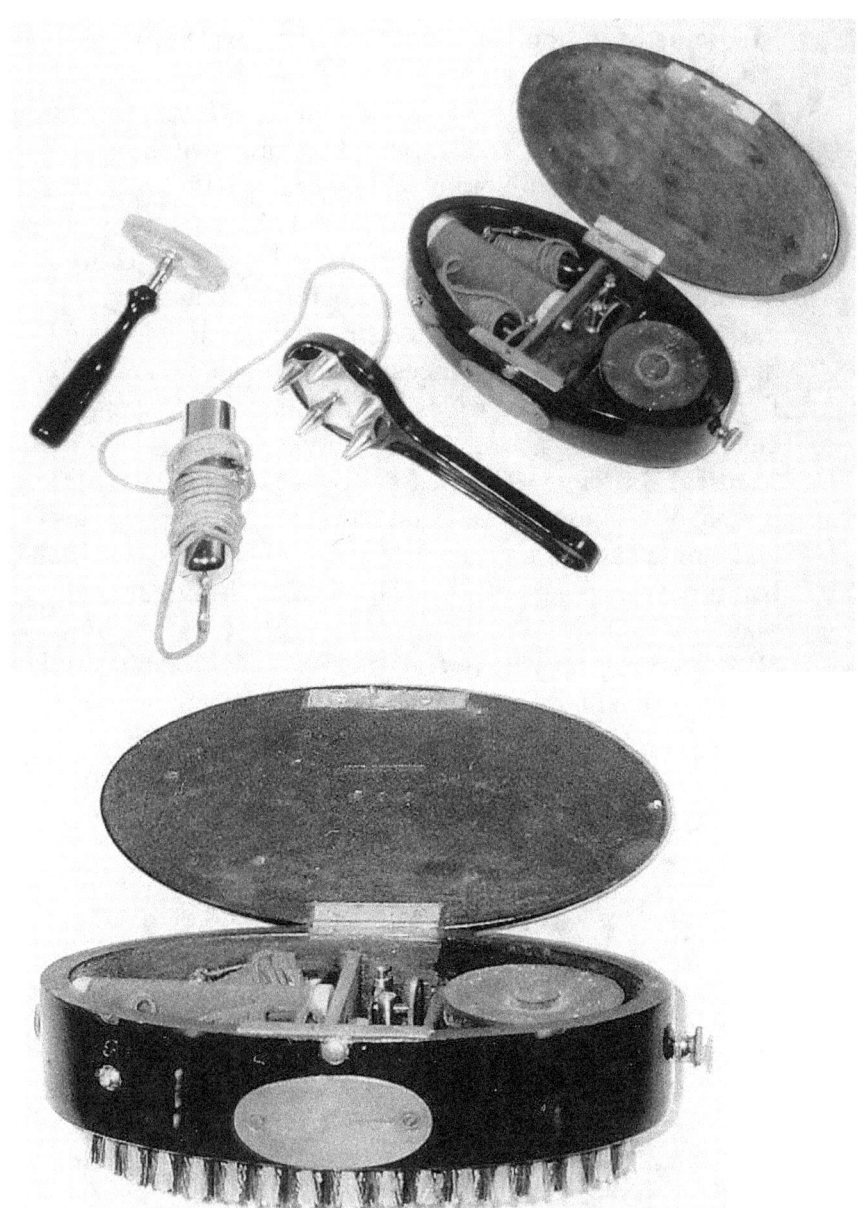

Personal faradic battery hair brush and scalp massage

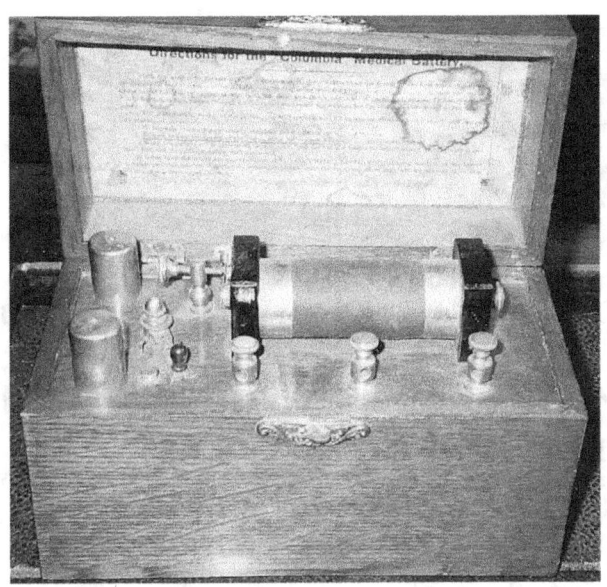

Pilling-Made Philadelphia Battery George P. Pilling and Son Company; Philadelphia, PA (9" x 5" x 5.5")

Portable Double Cell Faradic Battery Induction coil in oak wood box with hinged lid containing accessory compartment, 8.75" x 6.25" x 8.25".
Portable Faradic Battery Induction coil apparatus in oak wood box, hinged lid, nickel-plated hardware, 8.75"x6.25"x8".
Portable Faradic Battery (C.P. Pilling and Son) Induction coil apparatus in cherry wood box, angled front hinged lid, nickel-plated hardware, mirror-finish grounding electrode mounted inside front lid, 5.5" x 5.5" x 9.75".
Princess Mahogany carrying case with hinged lid and double side doors, various accessories, battery operated.

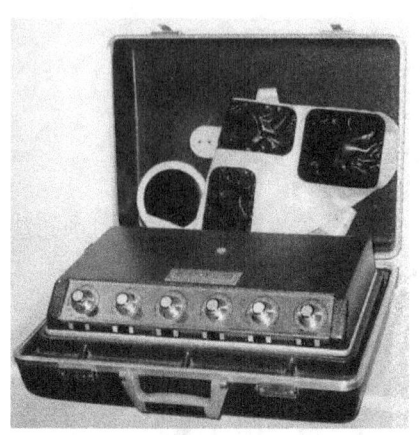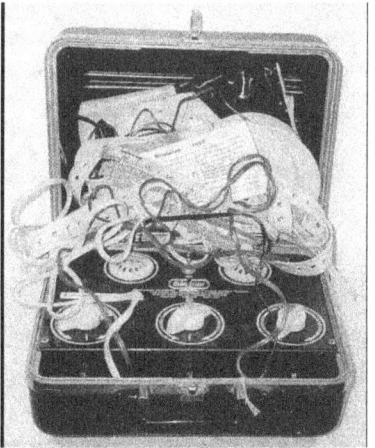

Relax-A-Cizor shock machines to stimulate muscles (1949-70), with body pads.

Rogers Consolidated Medical Apparatus Induction coil in cherry wood box, hinged lid contains accessories; 8.5"x5"x5.25".

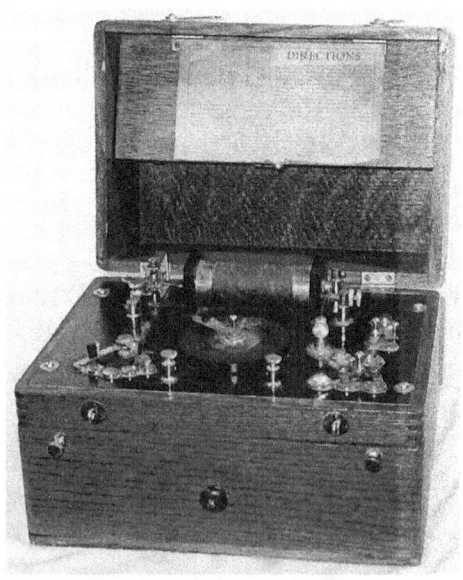

Sears-Roebuck Faradic Battery with rotary spark gap (11" x 8.75" x 8")

Seymour shock machine Oak wood box with nickel-plated hardware.
Stimulator (1995) Modified pushbutton, gas-grill igniter; press plunger to get shock to stimulate pain-blocking response.
Thermo Ozone Battery (1920s) Hinged-lid box containing glass vials, metal tube, disc electrodes, and strap-on contact pads.

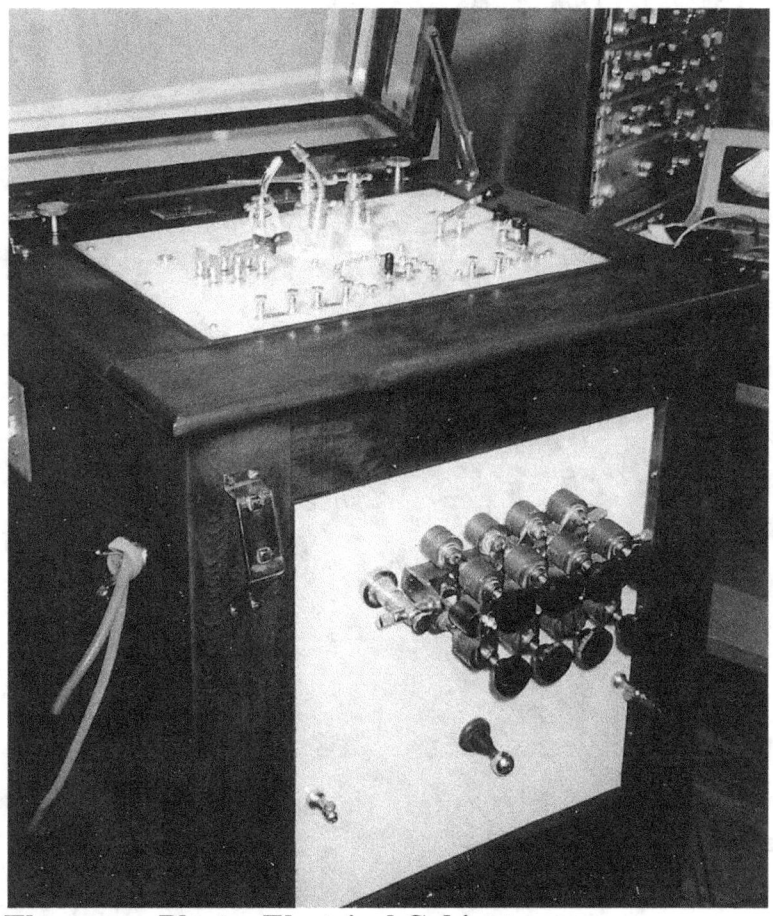

Thompson Plaster Electrical Cabinet

Voltamp Battery No. 4 "Samaritan" and No. 6 "Majestic" Induction coil apparatus in cherry wood box, hinged lid, latched black panel lifts to expose accessories, 8.25" x 5.25" x 5".

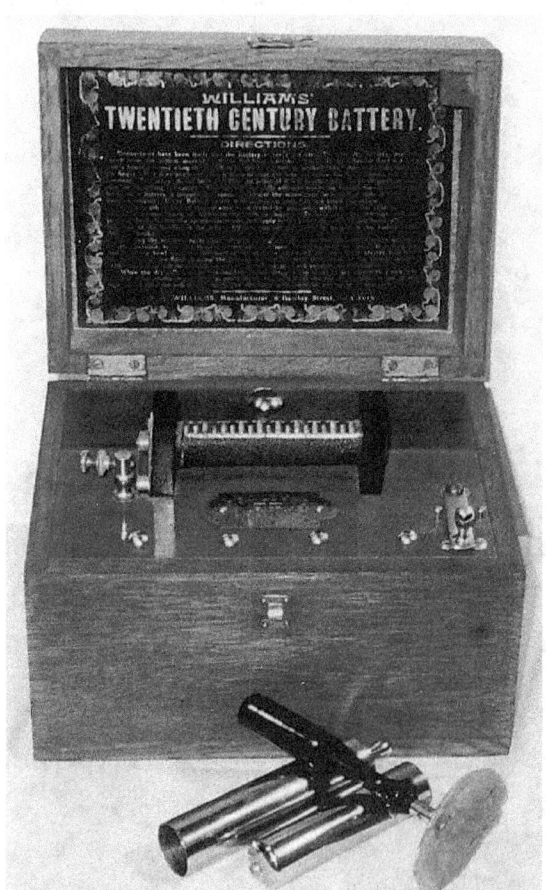

Williams Twentieth Century Battery (7.75" x 6" x 5.75")

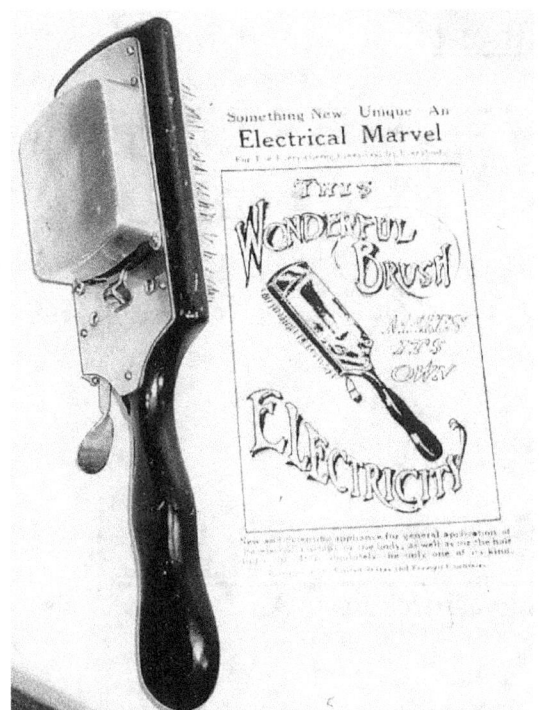

Wonder Brush Black wooden handle, steel bristles, thumb-operated magneto.

Electric equipment

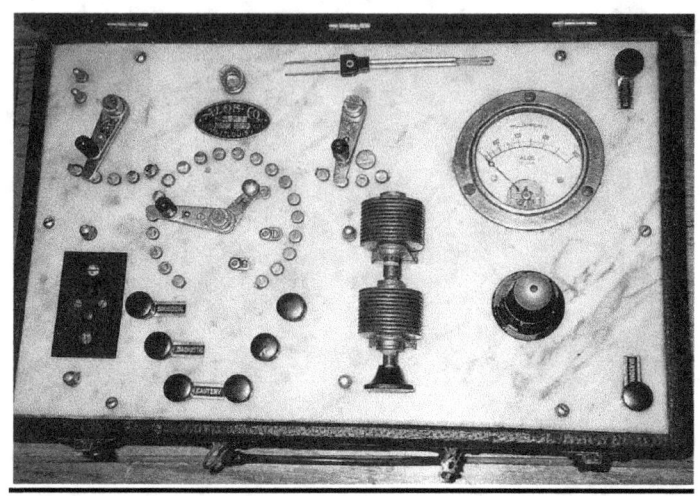

Aloe Sinusoidal/diagnostic/cautery Aloe Co., St. Louis, MO (17"x 11" x8")

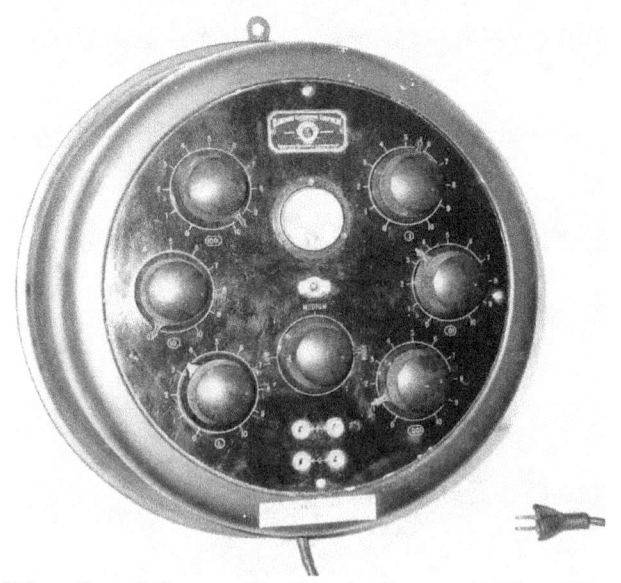

Blanchard Super Radionic Surge (17" x 7")

Beautypower device; white plastic case, gold grill, knob
Dr. Scott's Electric Corset and Belt $1-$3 in 1905.
Dr. Scott's Electric Tooth brush (1880s) charged with electromagnetic current to promote healthy teeth and gums.
Dynatone
Electropad

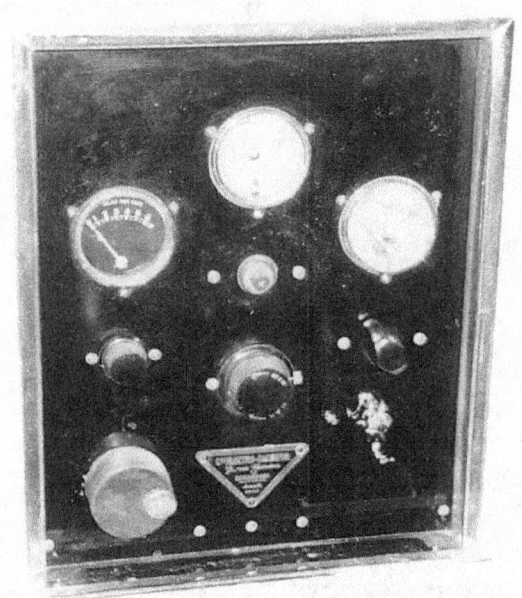

Electro-Salvator (Manufactured in France)

Fisher Type FO machine Mahogany box, 26" x 26" x 51" porcelain front, glass lift top, attachments.

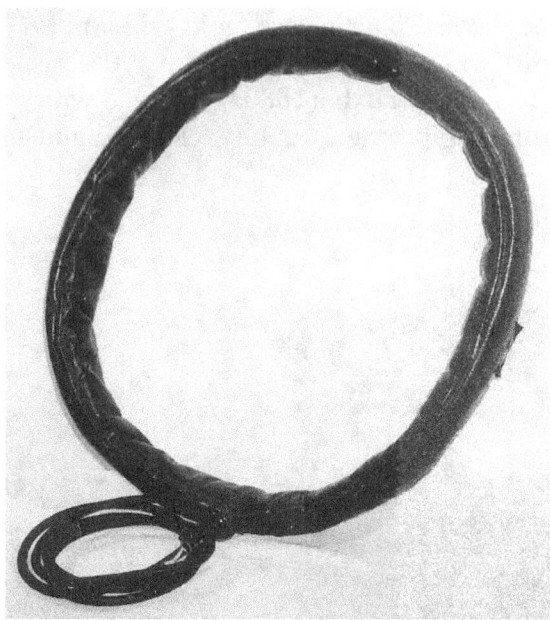

I-ON-A-CO (Wilshire Ring, 1925 by Gaylord Wilshire) increases cellular oxidation by magnetizing the iron in the blood; 18" diameter insulated-wire ring placed around the waist, with AC plug; demonstrates power by inductively illuminating a flashlight bulb connected to a small coil.

Overbeck's Rejuvenator Designed for consumers to treat a wide range of ailments by applying two tubular electrodes to the afflicted part of the body.
Theronoid (1928) Similar to the Wilshire I-ON-A-CO; wire coil plugged into an AC receptacle; demonstrated radiant energy by inductively lighting a flashlight bulb connected to a small loop of wire; cured variety of diseases and senility.

Wisconsin Oxygenator
Wonder Electric Generator

Electronic equipment

Atomotrone Cancer cure device (Dr. William M. Estep); wooden cabinet containing old radio set with colored tubes.

Auto Sweep Resonator III Combination Hieronymus, radionics, TENS device which automatically kills insect infestations in a field which has its photograph placed into it; also relaxes muscles and transmits subconscious messages to others.

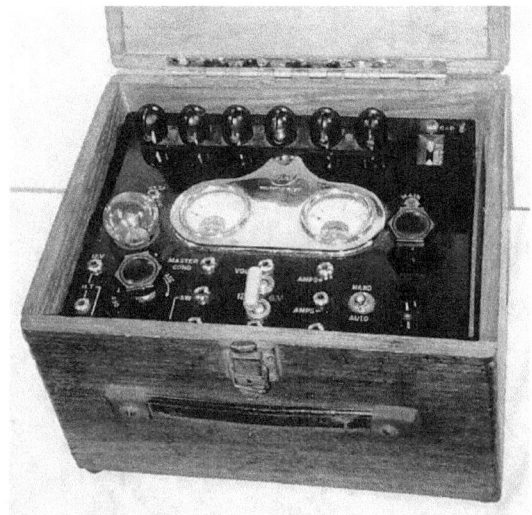

British Eagle Industries (11" x 8" x 9") nicknamed "The Pink Mouse" (No, I don't know why!)

Calbro Magnowave Radionic machine Black panel, two meters, 52 rheostats, 34 toggle switches, gold legends, oak roll-top secretary desk, 56" x 24" x 52".

Depolaray (1920s-1940s; Dr. Albert Abrams' Electronic Medical Foundation) Electromagnetic device.

Dermatron (1970s, Dr. Rheinhold Voll)

Diapulse (1970) Diathermy device.

Electro-Metabograph Made in Detroit by Ace Tool and Die; 3 black panels in an oak cabinet; loaded with dials; only 25 were ever made.

Electronic Magnetic Model G Suitcase unit containing a panel with switches, dials, pushbuttons, electrode terminals and lights; internal RF oscillator and amplifier for detecting and emitting radio waves.

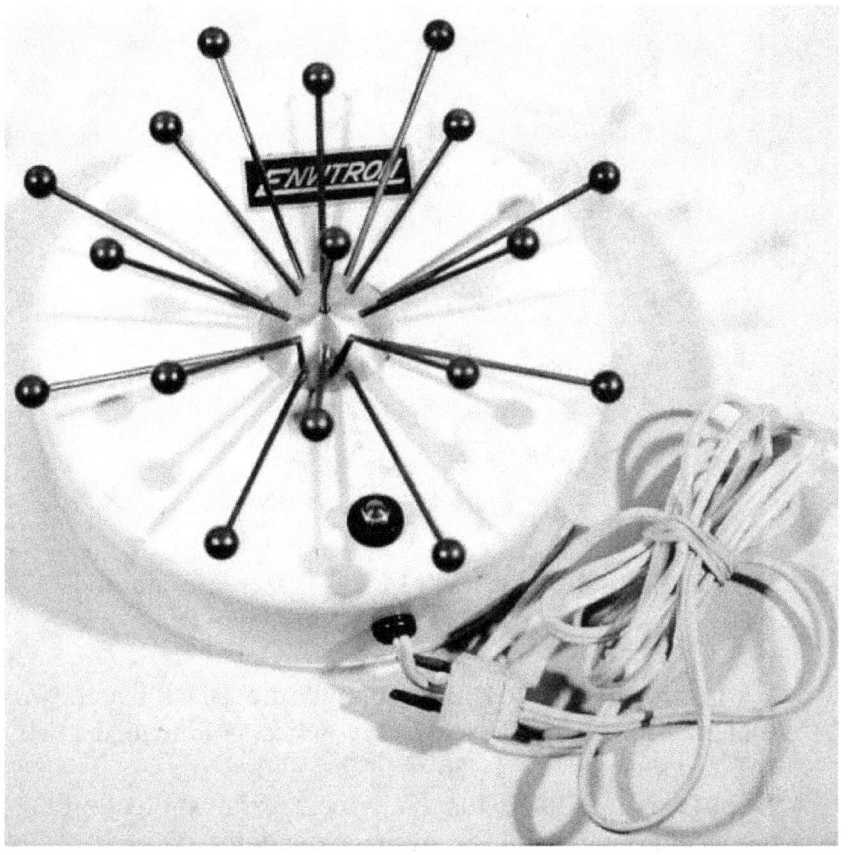

Envitron electric field generator

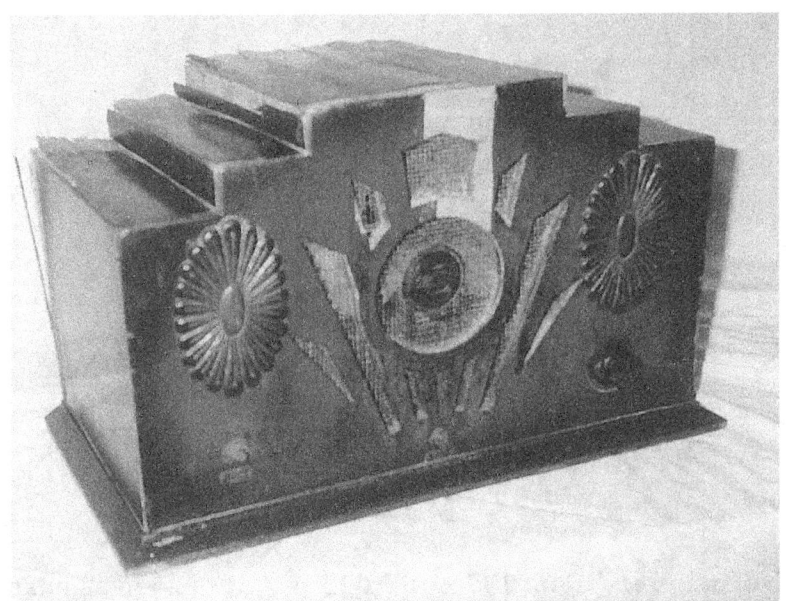

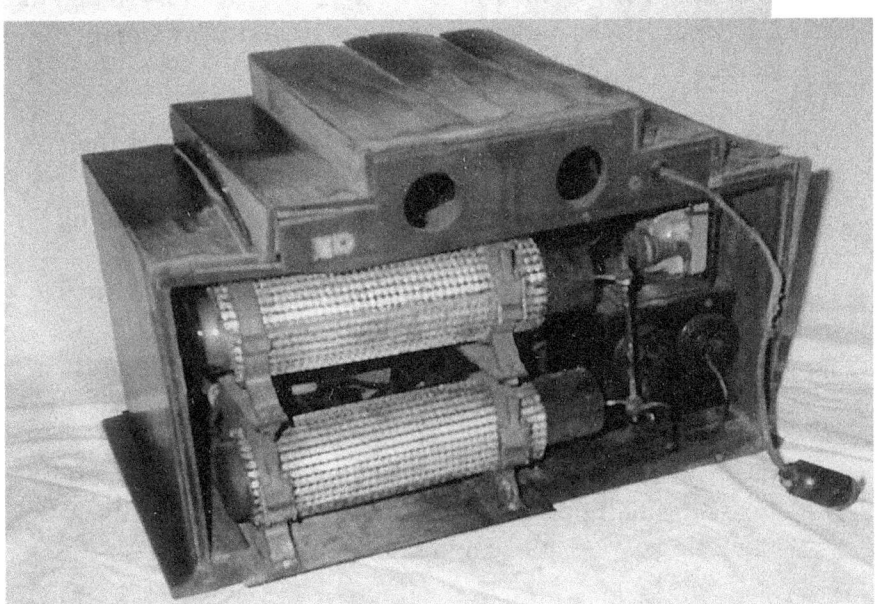

Fanozone (1930s) Ozone generator in a wooden Art Deco, radio-style case with two high-voltage coils, transformer, and fan.

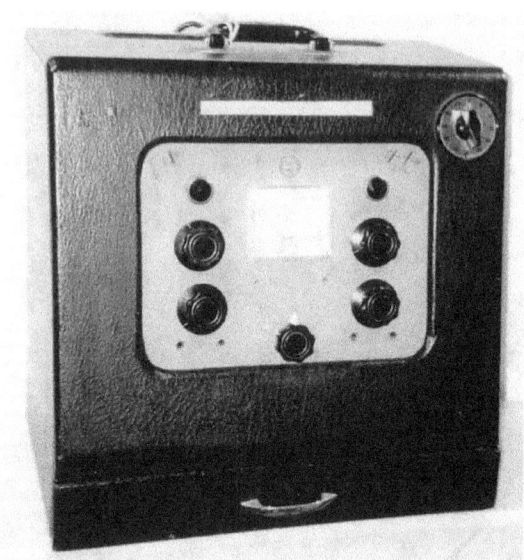

Harmonizer (1966; 19" x 19" x 13") AM radio in a guitar case that moves a meter and sends audio to "treatment" connectors.

Health-Aire Ozone ion generator, white plastic, grilled front   .
Interro (1980s, Dr. F. Fuller Royal) Generates whining noise, single probe, scale on computer screen.
MacGregor Rejuvenator (1920s) Bed with cylindrical shroud paneled with dials and gauges; generated radio waves and ultraviolet radiation to reverse the aging process.
NatureTronics Model D Rife generator (2006, $2000) Ggenerates hundreds of discrete radio frequencies to destroy viruses, bacteria and fungi causing nearly every disease; small portable instrument with LED readouts, numeric keypad, pulse and intensity controls.

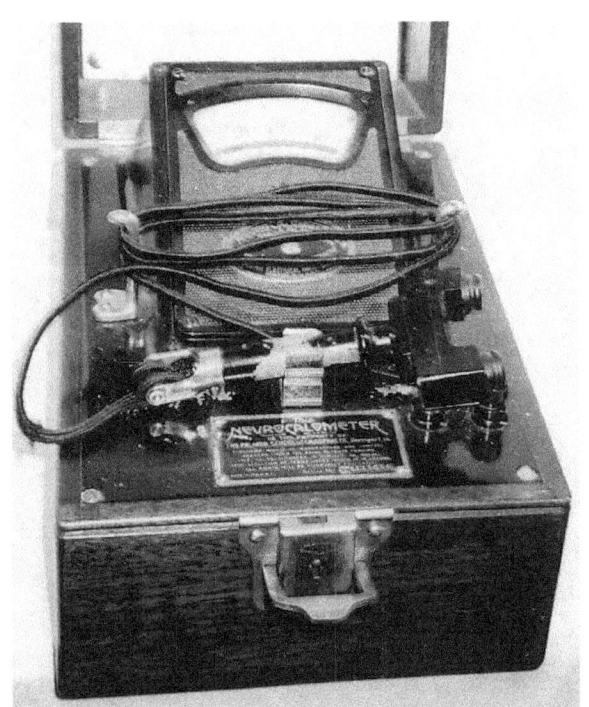

Neurocalometer (7" x 7.75" x 10.5")

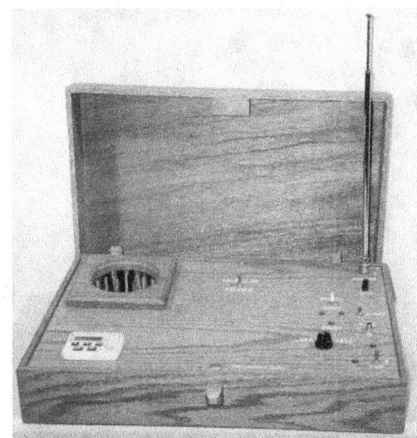

Neutralize/Balance (no identification; (18" x 12" x 5")

Neurolinometer

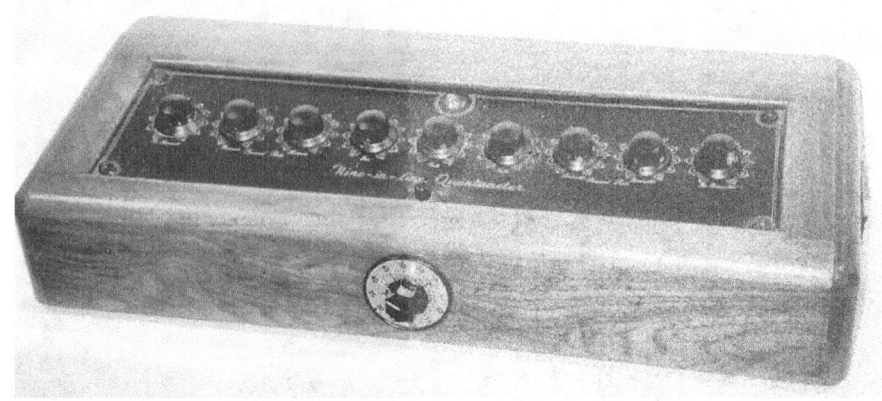

Nine-In-Line Q Quantumeter (26" x 6" x 10")

Oscillotron
Pathosine Wood and metal console therapeutic device
with dials, switches, lights and plug outlets for electrodes
and pads; intended to measure and perform therapy to eyes
and muscles.

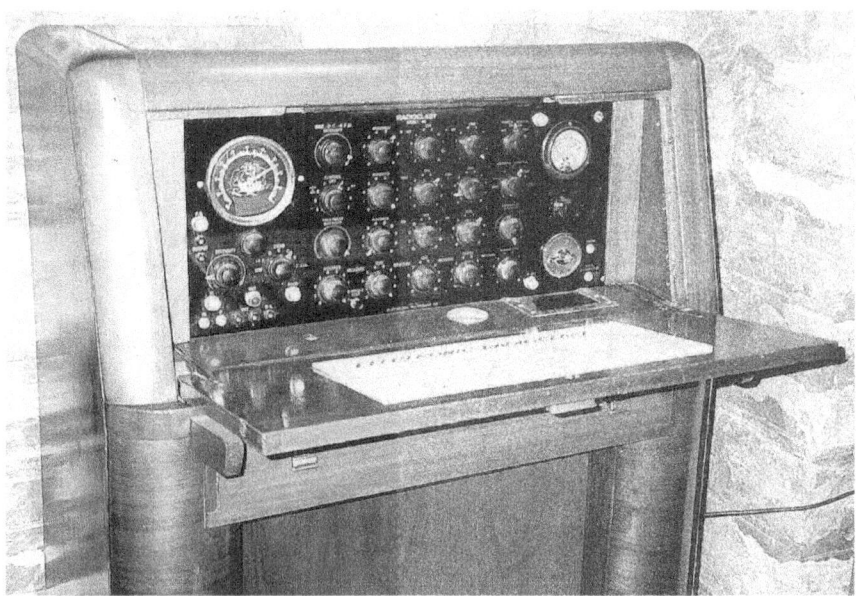

Radio-Clast model 40 (36" x 44" x 18")

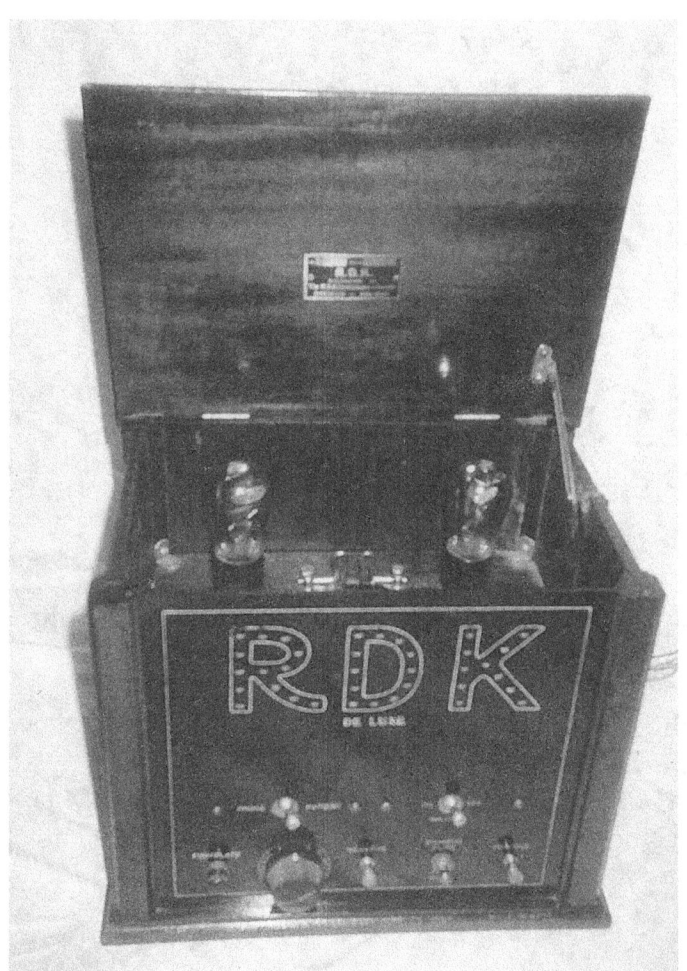

RDK short wave apparatus (1929) Bakelite panel, wood box with hinged lid, glass probe, two 201A vacuum tubes; 15-watt red, green, blue light bulbs rear-illuminate the RDK.

Nemectron

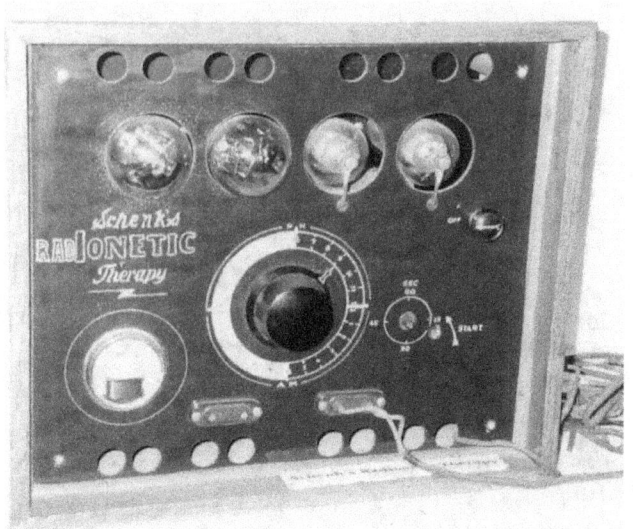

Schenk's Radionetic Therapy (15" x 13" x 10")

Shoe-fitting fluoroscope (1940s-60s) Wood-cabinet Xray console with upper viewing ports for customer and salesman to see foot bones in new shoes; by the 1970s, outlawed in the U.S.
Short Wave Oscillotron
Tricho/Hair-X hair remover (1925, Albert Geyser, M.D.) Wood cabinet with projecting, cylindrical, metal drum containing X-ray tube.

Radioactive products

Bioray (1930; William J.A. Bailey) Small container
ostensibly radiating therapeutic gamma rays.

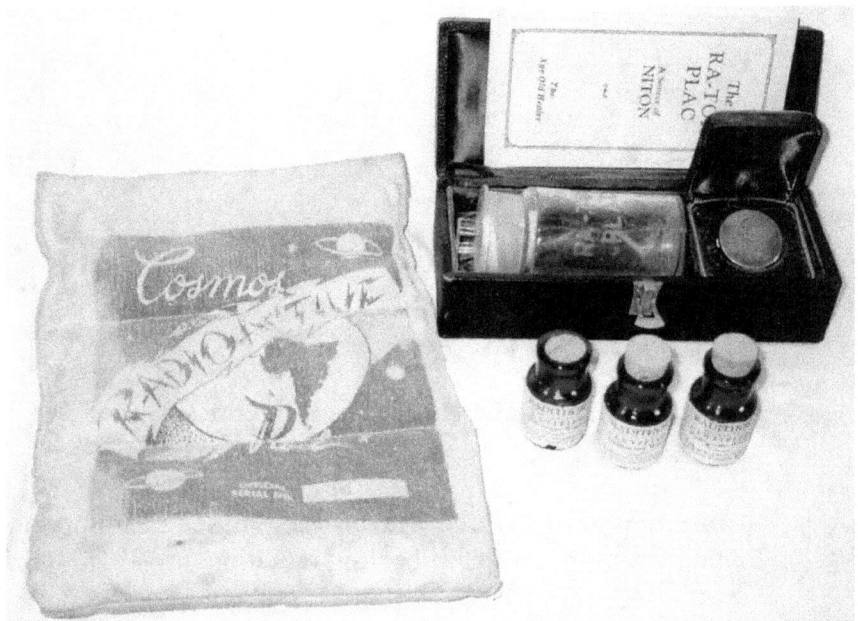

Cosmos Bag (1928) Bag of crushed uranium ore; radiation
would relieve arthritis, sinusitis, asthma and other
maladies; and RA-TON PLAC, "A source of NITON, the
age-old healer."

Radioendocrinator (1930; American Endocrine
Laboratories, William J.A. Bailey, Ward Leathers)
Decorative box contains 2" x 3" x 0.4" metal-box and
radioactive substance to achieve metabolic balance of the
endocrine gland.

Radithor (1920s) Half-ounce bottles of radioactive liquid
to energize depleted organs.

Rator-Lac (1920s) Home kit to make radioactive tonic;
fill bottle with water and set it on the radioactive disc.

Thoronator (1930; William J.A. Bailey) Small glass vial containing cylinder emitting "thoron."

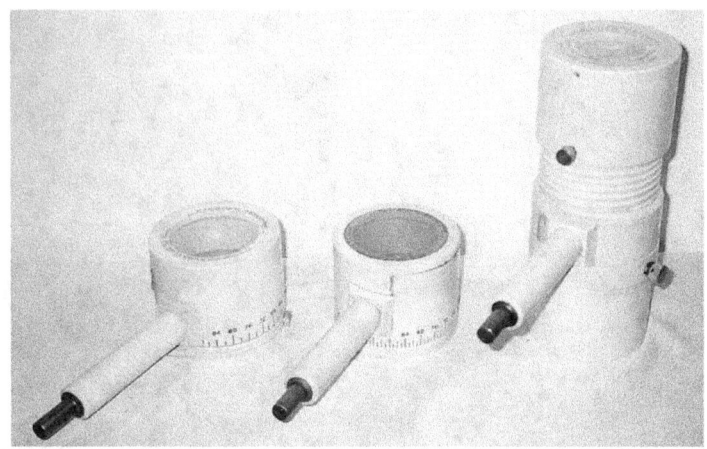

Toftness Chiropractic Radiation Detector (4" x 3.5" x 12")

Uranium Wonder Glove Gravel-filled mitten claiming to contain uranium or to emit healing radiation.

Lights

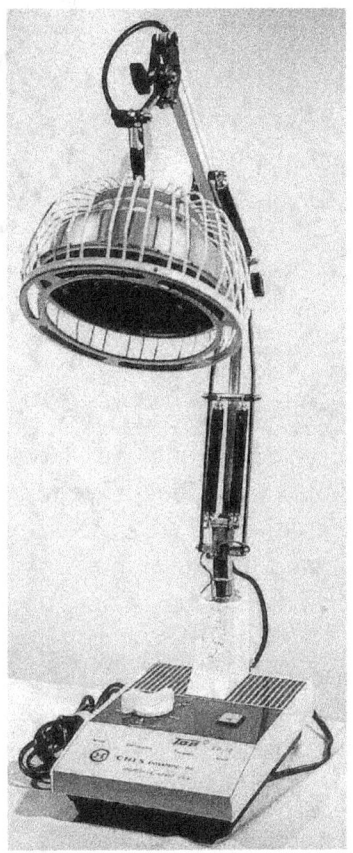

Chi's Enterprise TOP Far-infrared heat lamp with a wide range of cure claims

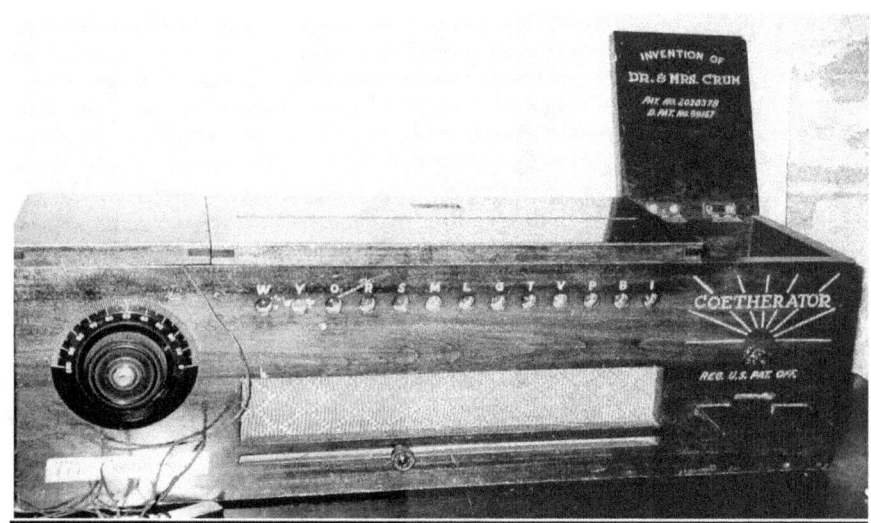

Coetherator (1926; invention of Dr. and Mrs. Crum) Rheostat and sliding light bulb passed behind lettered apertures which could cure all diseases, regrow amputated fingers, remove iron from a well, provide financial treatments, and kill all insects in a farmer's field up to 70 miles away.

Color-Therm (1940s) Wood cabinet or black patent leather carrying case containing intertwined neon tubes for feet to touch, and a cord to a hand-held, U-shaped, neon wand to massage the body; retarded aging, cured any disease.

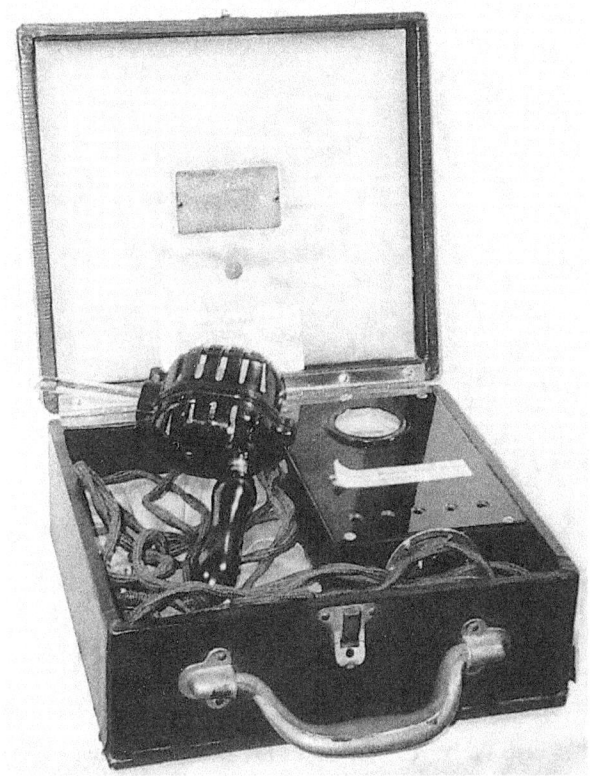

Comp-Sol-Lite (MacGregor Corporation' 11.25" x 5" x 10.25") Ordinary, incandescent, light bulb which was said to emit enough UV radiation to cure a variety of afflictions.

Curay Lamp (See Comp-Sol-Lite)
Hair growing helmet (1940s) Aluminum bowl, containing Christmas tree bulb and electric cord.
Radionics machine (1921, L. Ron Hubbard) Box containing tiny, colored lights for diagnosis.
Radioscope (1920s-1930s; Dr. Albert Abrams "Radionics") Oak cabinet with dials and glowing lights, to diagnose disease by scanning drops of blood with radio waves.

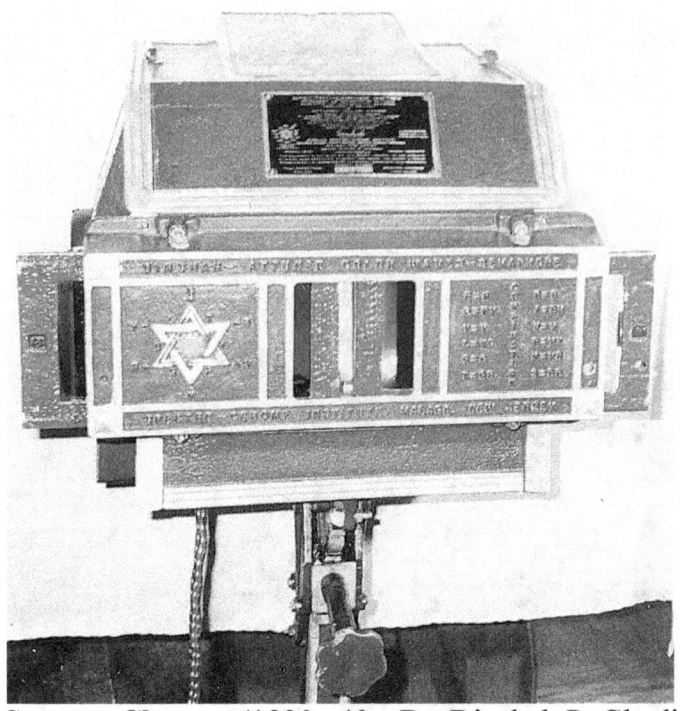

Spectro-Chrome (1930s-40s; Dr. Dinshah P. Ghadiali)
Cast aluminum, 1000W bulb, water tank, colored glass
filters; cure-all.

Visible Color Spectrum Projector (See Spectro-Chrome)
Patient sits nude in the dark, facing north, and stares at the
light during certain phases of the moon.

Diagnostic devices

Accupath 1000 (1970s, Dr. Rheinhold Voll)

Advanced Bio-Photon Integrator (1990s) Automated radionics instrument tunes in on the subject's energetic mineral base by analyzing his aura every 40 seconds and creates homeopathic/isopathic remedies.

Amalgameter (1991) Detects by electrical current the most offensive silver fillings for removal.

Anapathic automatic scan-treat (T. Galen Hieronymus, Advanced Sciences Research And Development Corp.) Diagnoses and treats symptoms through a vial of water.

Cardiolectameter Model H Wood console diagnostic and therapeutic device with switches, rheostat, meters and a speaker which emitted sound representing circulatory pressure.

Cambridge Electrocardiograph machine (1930)

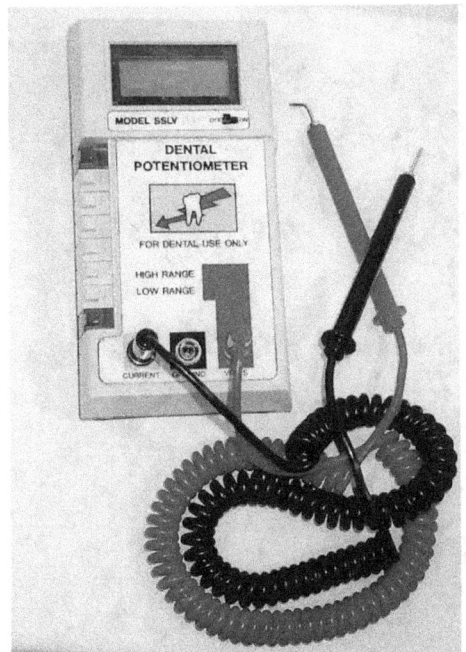

Dental Potentiometer – modern quackery

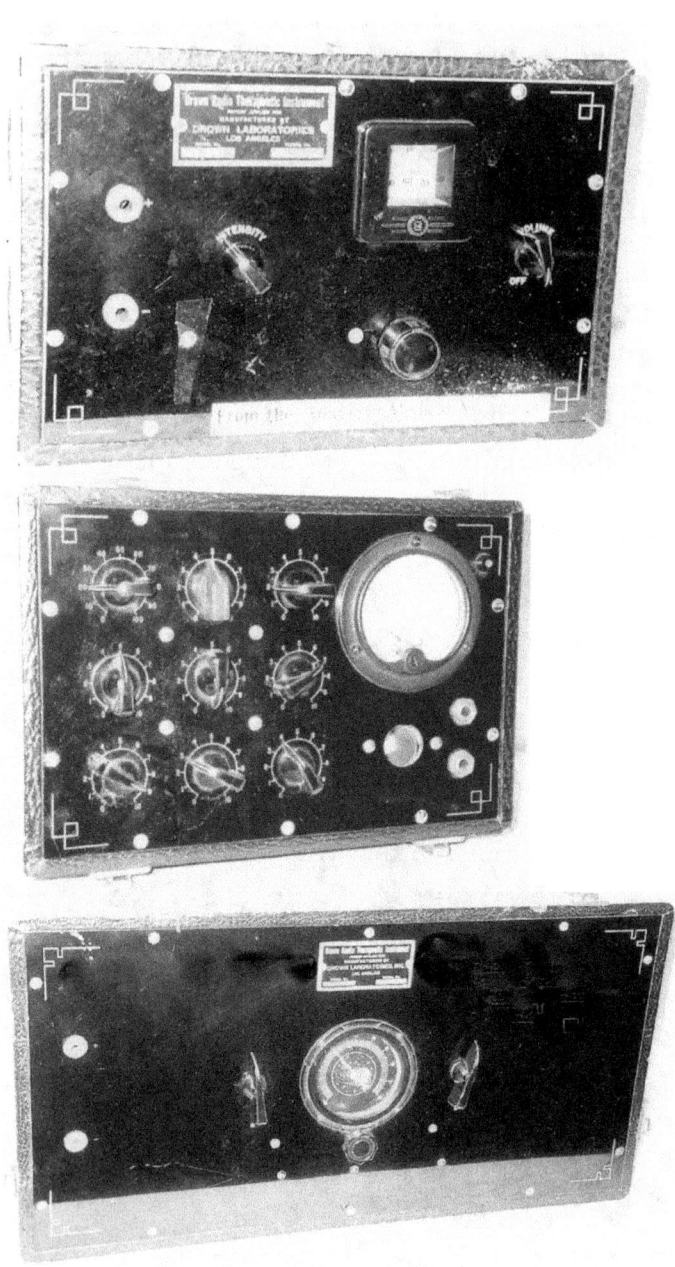

Drown Radio Therapeutic Instrument (Model 30, sections 1 and 2)
(1920s-40s; Dr. Ruth B. Drown, chiropractor and osteopath); diagnostic instruments. Model 30 is a black-textured box with 9 knobs and meter on top Bakelite panel; two internal dissimilar-metal blocks wired to two external metal-plate electrodes. Place a drop of blood on a blotter, tune in on distant patient's radio frequency to broadcast treatment.

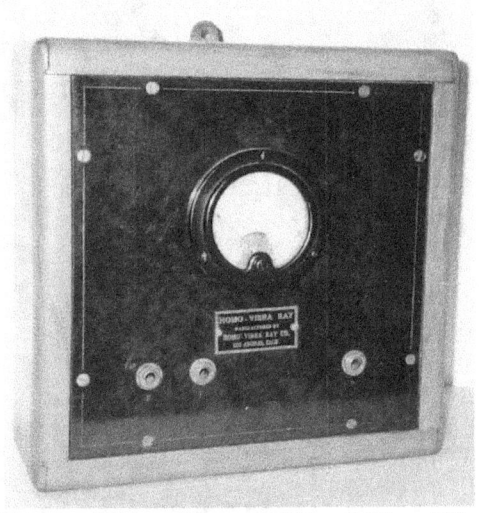

Homo Vibra Ray (10" x 10" x 4")

Dynamizer Dr. Abrams's short, cylindrical, diagnostic apparatus to test blood samples for "radioactivity." See "Oscilloclast."
Electro Ion-A-Meter, **Model A** Black panel with 3 jacks, large rheostat dial, earphones and electrodes, black leatherette case with corner reinforcers, accessories in hinged lid, 11.5" x 7" x 8.25"; diagnostic instrument listening for AC hum as body is rubbed with probes.

Electrodiagnostic devices (1950s, Dr. Rheinhold Voll) Galvanometer, with one brass and one gauze-covered probe.

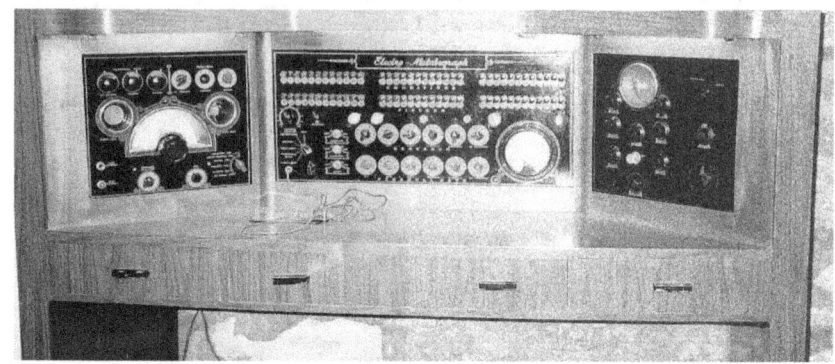

Electro Metabograph
Made by Ace Tool and Die, Chicago, IL; Only 25 of these consoles were ever manufactured

Electropsychometer; "E-Meter" (1950s-1960s; L. Ron Hubbard, Dianetics, Church of Scientology).

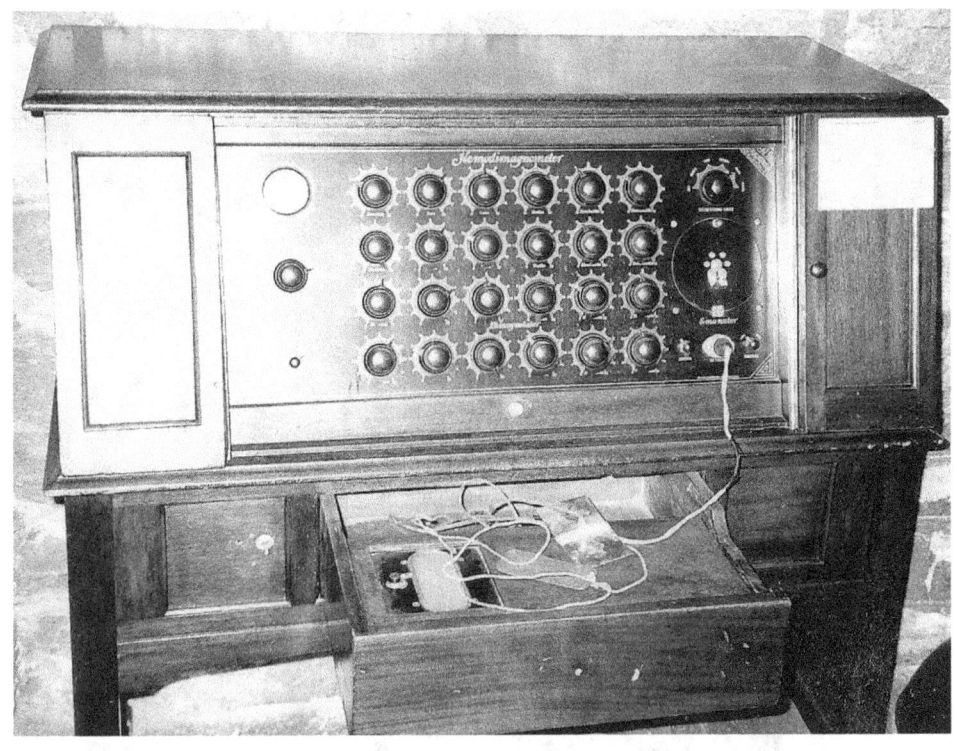

Hemodimagnometer (1940s) Diagnostic machine wired
to a piece of metal pressed against the forehead of a healthy
person; insert a drop of blood, or an autograph of the
patient, and tap the healthy person's abdomen to find a
vibratory frequency for patient's cure.

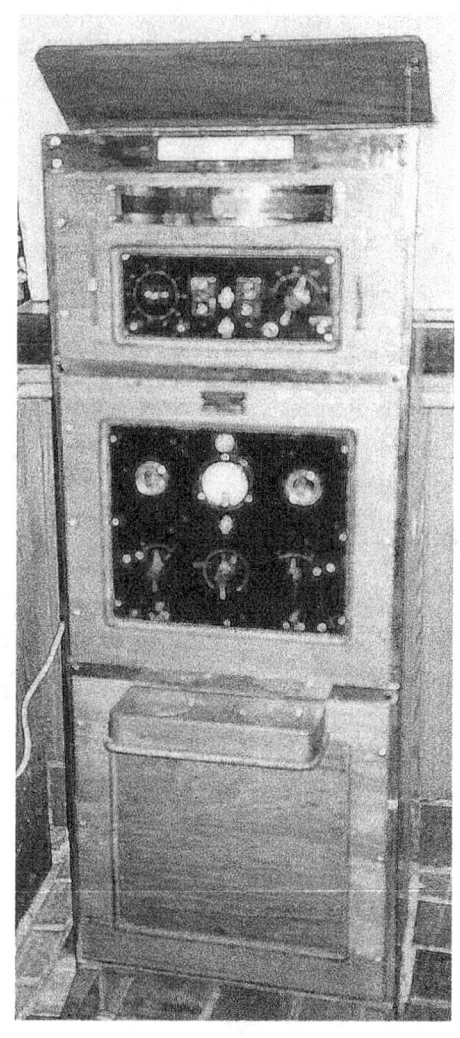

Micro-Dynameter diagnostic machine, model A (1950s, F.C. Ellis)

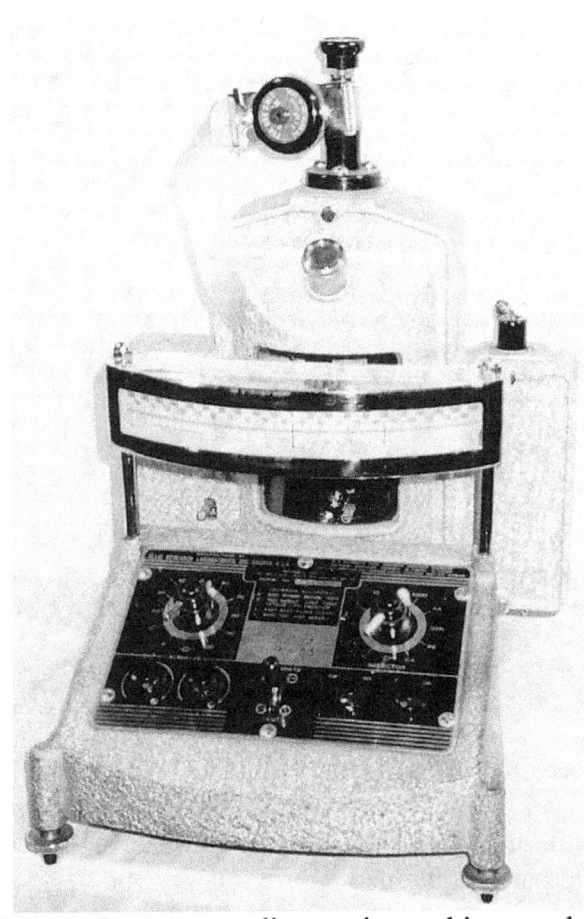

Micro-Dynameter diagnostic machine, model SA-1 (1950s, F.C. Ellis) Desktop, textured, die-cast cabinet, six knobs and toggle switch operate high-sensitivity galvanometer with electrodes.

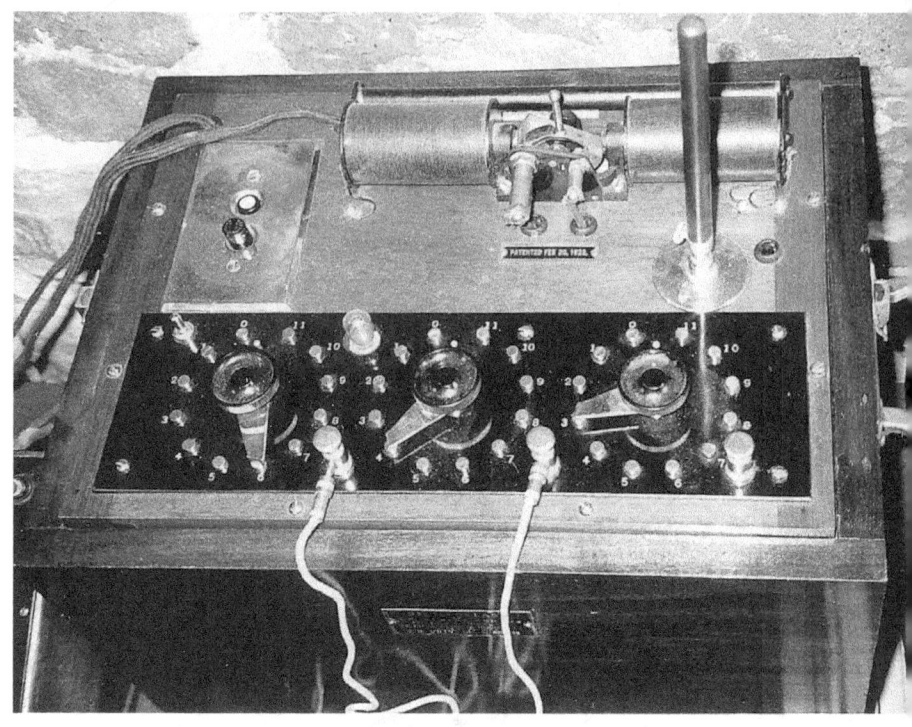

Oscilloclast machine (1916-1920s, Dr. Albert Abrams, Electronic Medical Foundation; by 1923, 44 manufacturers were making similar models) Desk console model with drop-down front panel contained approximately 100 unconnected switches and knobs for diagnosis and treatment. Portable version (shown here) consisted of a wooden box with side handles, electric wires attached to a cold-water pipe, a wooden rotary switchbox ("rheostatic dynamizer"), and a short, cylindrical "Dynamizer" ("condenser") for receiving dried blood, urine, saliva, or a signature; included was a disc on a small handle ("brow electrode") to place against the forehead.

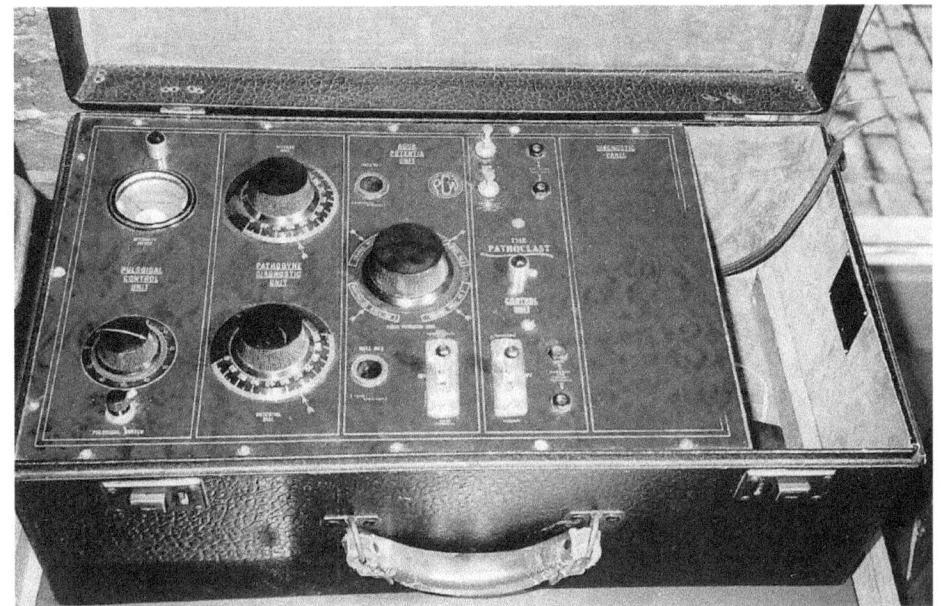

Pathoclast machine (Abrams; 22" x 9" x 11.5")

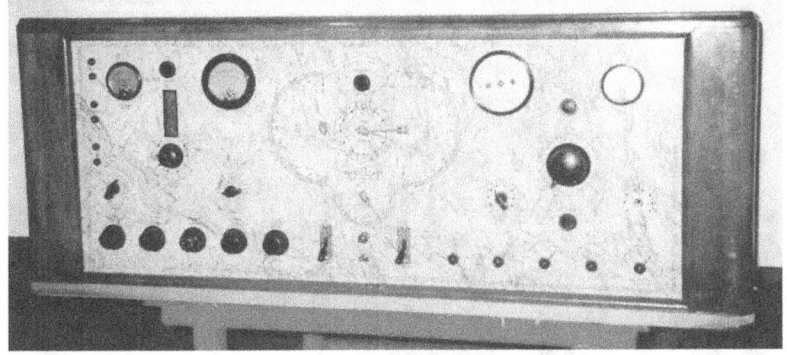

Pathoclast machine (18.75" x 14.5" x 8"; 1920s; Dr Arles Pottle, Dayton, OH; distributed by Pathometric Laboratories, Chicago, IL). Desk console, diagnostic and therapeutic device with a variety of meters, knobs, dials, switches, lights, and specimen wells to measure the electrical vibrations from the body and reradiate similar radiations from the electrodes to the body.

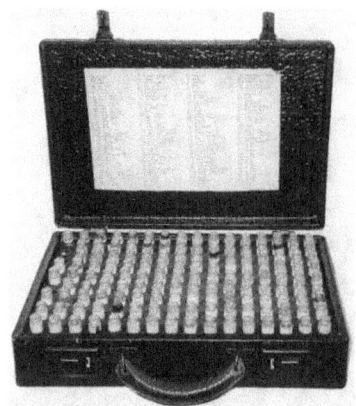

Pathoclast Allergen Phials

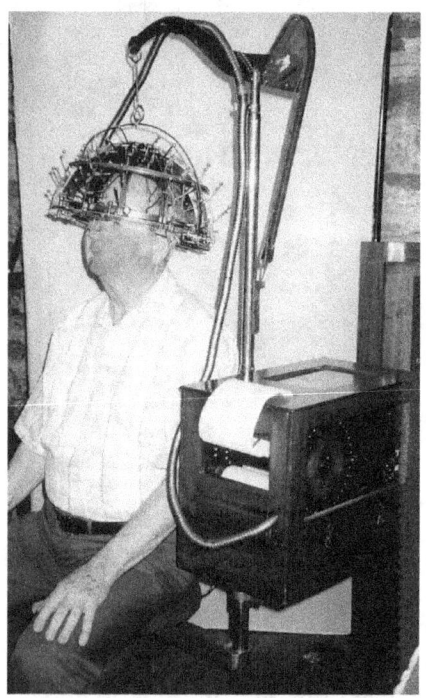

Psychograph (1931-1935, Henry Lavery) Metal phrenology helmet for measuring character traits; 32 adjustable feelers connected by cable to recording box/printer; included nickel-plated stand and padded seat.

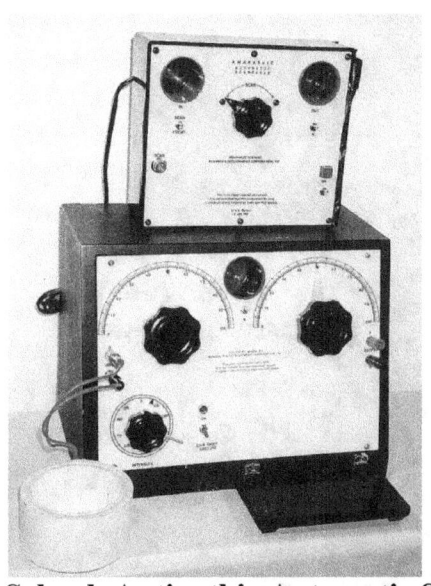

Schenk Antipathic Automatic Scan-Test (Advanced Sciences Research and Development Corporation; 2 pieces: 8.5" x 7" x 3" and 13" x 9.75" x 8")

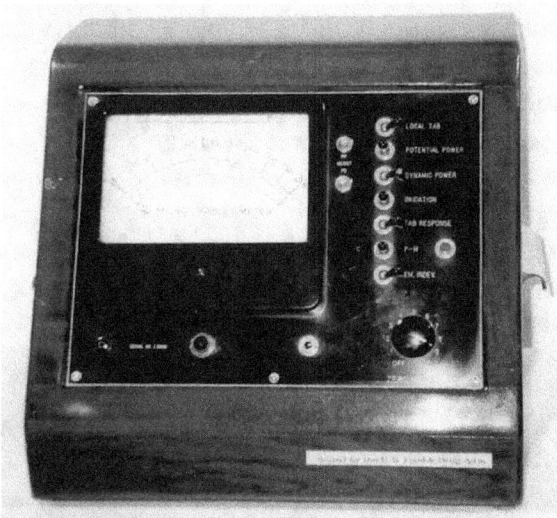

Schenk's Micro-Tabulometer (15" x 13" x 11")

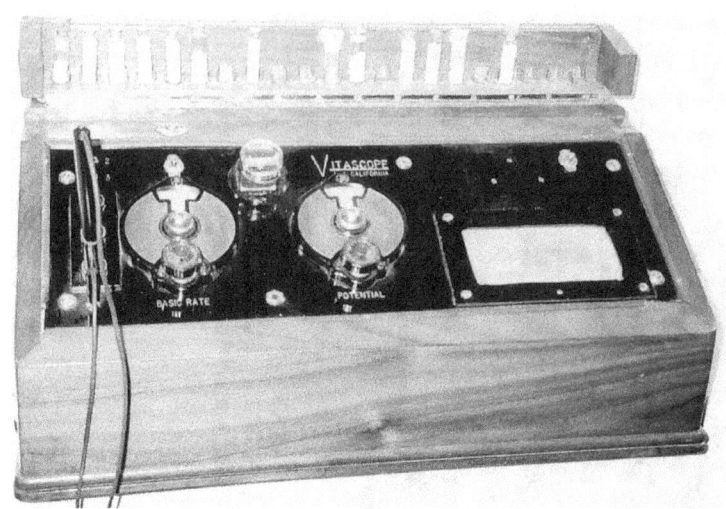

Vitascope (23" x 9" x 12.5")

Wish Machine II radionics/psychotronics tachyon thoughtform amplifier (1998, $710) Customer places a photograph between two copper plates and thinks about what they want: success, money, love, or angel contact. **Toftness Radiation Detector**; (1970s, Irwing N. Toftness) Chiropractic plastic cylinder containing plastic lenses, rubbed up and down the spine to detect "resistance."

Heating elements
DeAns Infra Red Therapeutic Mittens Electrically-heated mittens powered by AC cord; "treatment for arthritis, rheumatism and nervous conditions."

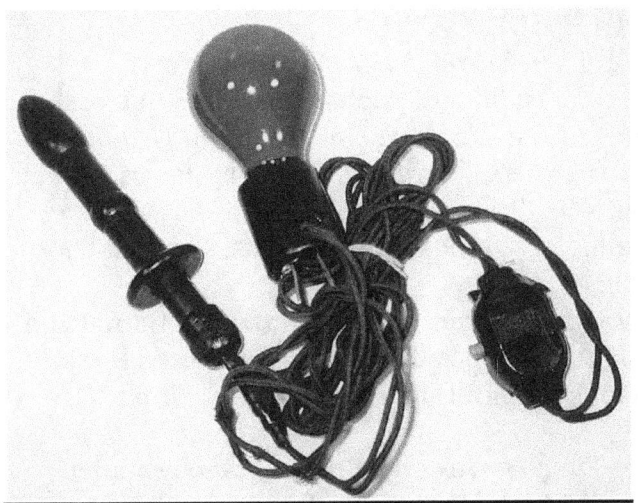

G-H-R Electric Thermitis Dilator (1918) Foot-long, phallus-shaped, rectal probe connected by twisted-pair cord to light bulb assembly and AC plug; inserted into the rectum to "excite the abdominal brain" by warming the prostate gland to restore sexual energy and cure other diseases.

Magneto-conservative Insoles (1900, Wilson/Actina Appliance) Magnets to keep the feet warm.
Prostate Gland Warmer (See G-H-R, above)
Thermalaid (Electro Thermal Co.) Rectally-inserted plastic probe cures prostate disorders and hemorrhoids.
Urbeteit's Sinuothermic machine (1940s)

WEB PAGE RESOURCES
http://www.museumofquackery.com
http://www.quackwatch.org/
http://www.quackwatch.org/13Hx/TM/12.html
(Excellent article with exhaustive reference list)
http://www.fda.gov/ForConsumers/ProtectYourself/
HealthFraud/default.htm
http://www.consumer.ftc.gov/topics/health-fitness

REFERENCE PUBLICATIONS

The Golden Age of Quackery by Stewart H. Holbrook, a compendium of pitchmen and their pitches.

Medical Messiahs: A Social History of Health Quackery in Twentieth-Century America, by James Harvey Young; Rev. 1992, Princeton University Press. An excellent chronology of nostrums, gadgets, and their court histories.

The Health Robbers, edited by Stephen Barrett and William T. Jarvis, Published 1993 by Prometheus Books, 59 John Glenn Drive, Buffalo, NY 14228-2197; ph. 716-837-2475.

Four White Horses and a Brass Band by Violet "Lotus Blossom" McNeal, the colorful and tawdry autobiography of one of America's greatest pitch women.

Pink Pills for Pale People by F.W. Saul

Step Right Up by Brooks McNamara, a history of the American medicine shows.

Nostrums and Quackery by Arthur J. Cramp, MD. Three successive volumes in early 20th century: Volume 1, 1911; volume 2, 1921; volume 3, 1936. A comprehensive look at medical quackery in its finest hour, with biting commentary and court histories.

Sears-Roebuck catalog reprints before 1936.

The Great American Fraud by Samuel Hopkins Adams, Colliers *The American* Weekly, Oct. 7, 1905-Sept. 1906 (reprinted later by the AMA as a book). This singular, most devastating assault against medical quackery led to the Pure Food and Drug Act.

Vi-Ton-Ka Medicine Show; Glenn Hinson, NY American Place Theater, 1984 (pamphlet).

Notices of Judgement published by the FDA, U.S. Dept of Agriculture (Department of Chemistry pre-WW II).